CW00692443

Know Your Colour Personality

Revised edition

Alison Standish

Theresa Sundt

Illustrations by Theresa Sundt

First published 2014
Revised edition 2017

ISBN 978-0-9558669-7-5

Cover design by Theresa Sundt
Typeset by Helius
www.helius.co.uk

Printed in the UK by One Digital

Contents

Introduction

We are all very interested in who we are and how we interact with each other on this planet. Many books, films, workshops and courses are available to help us understand ourselves and others better.

In our original book, we combined the ancient art of colour therapy with up-to-date, 21st-century concepts of colour personalities, and created a fun and interesting look at how different colour personalities interact. We decided to write this book together for the following reasons:

- We found that we both had a passion and love of colour, and have invested time and energy into studying colour over the last 15 years. We have given many hundreds of insightful and very helpful readings into the relevance of peoples' colour personalities, and now wish to share our knowledge with you.
- We have discovered how colour helps us to make beneficial differences in our lives, and we have been able to positively transform our relationships with ourselves, our family, partners, friends and work colleagues.
- We have been able to introduce colour into our own homes and working environments and those of others, to enhance the positive aspects of these relationships.

To provide as much information as possible in this book, in Part 1 we created nine subdivisions in each colour personality chapter. We start with the colour personality's 'General traits', then 'Tricky traits', which alert about the weaker side of the personality. These are followed by 'Health and well-being', 'In the bedroom', 'In the family', 'At work',

'How best to handle the personality', 'Helpful hints for when things get tough' and 'Personality affirmation' (on how to strengthen the core of each colour personality).

When the weaker side of our personality takes over, sabotaging our peace and well-being, we need to consider our essence, which is our ideal state of being, and try to resonate with it. An archetypal illustration for each colour supports the colour personality's affirmation

In this new revised edition, we have added a second part of the book that focuses on our additional three colours in our overall colour chart. There is a unique colour for the day, month and year of birth. These are either known as 'supportive' colours or 'journey' colours, as they relate to childhood behaviour, day-to-day skills and life aspirations.

Along with the core colour personality, which is the most dominant part of our colour chart, interpreting and consciously applying the qualities of our day's, month's and year's colours will provide deeper guidance on how to become the best version of ourselves.

We radiate our personality's colours, and we are constantly interacting with other people's colours, which delight or mystify us. Colour with its own distinct language gives a fascinating and insightful view of not just our personal life journeys but that of family, friends and colleagues

The colour adventure that you are about to embark on has given us both the opportunities to grow and develop along with great 'Aha!' moments – we hope you enjoy them too!

Alison and Theresa
Gold and Magenta!

PART 1
Your colour personality

Colour and numbers

There are two decisive factors for our unique colour personality – a colour and a number.

Numbers have been respected for their mystical nature since ancient times. Numbers, similar to colours, have their own energy. Pythagoras wrote over 2,500 years ago about the nine numbers that he believed were profoundly mystical. He used the numbers 1–9 because 0 was not yet a concept in ancient Greece. He travelled to India and Egypt to expand his knowledge, and he wrote about several numerical systems used by those civilisations. The Pythagorean method, dating back to around 500 BC, stemmed from those writings and teachings. It became popular through Plato and his other students, and it is the method used most often by modern-day numerologists.

In the 1960s a method to categorise people into nine distinct groups of personalities was established. It was the result of a major study of different ancient systems, including the Pythagorean method, that help us to understand human nature.

The nine personality numbers acquired additional accuracy in describing the traits of each personality by the allocation of a different colour to each number. Each colour is linked to one of the energy centres of the human body, as in the well-established Ayuverdic tradition.

The nine-colour system can be extremely useful to all of us as a source of self-knowledge because it acts like a 'mirror', revealing features of our personality that are normally invisible to us.

Most of the time, people function habitually, as if on automatic pilot, according to their basic personality type. Usually, this allows us to get along well enough in our lives, but when our normal routine breaks down or the stresses of our lives increase too much, our normal ways of coping also tend to break down or become dysfunctional. By seeing clearly what our habitual patterns are – noticing what we are doing and why we are doing it, and at what cost to ourselves and others – we hold the key to our liberation. By knowing what our colour type is, we are able to see ourselves – to catch ourselves 'in the act' – as we move through the day. Learning about the ideal side of our personality, we are given clear directions on how to reach our potential within our abilities. With this increased self-awareness, we are also able to avoid reacting in potentially dangerous ways.

Calculating your personality

The colours that correspond to the nine personality numbers are:

1 = Red	4 = Green	7 = Violet
2 = Orange	5 = Blue	8 = Magenta
3 = Yellow	6 = Indigo	9 = Gold

To find the colour of a personality, you will need that person's date of birth. Start by adding together each number in the date of birth; and keep adding until you have a one-digit number. For example:

15/11/1965 = 1 + 5 (day), 1 + 1 (month), 1 + 9 + 6 + 5 (year)

1 + 5 + 1 + 1 + 1 + 9 + 6 + 5 = 29

2 + 9 = 11

1 + 1 = 2 = orange personality

You now have the core details of an individual's personality and the colour they vibrate on a day-to-day basis.

Calculate your core personality and that of your friends, family, colleagues and partners:

Are you the same colour as someone?
Are you the opposite colour to someone?
Are you a warm colour (red, orange or yellow) or are you cooler (blue, indigo or violet)?
Are you very grounded (red)?
Are you vibrating at a higher frequency (magenta or gold)?

There is no right or wrong, good or bad – just the colours as you see them.

We are more unique than just our core personality colour, so we can also use the colours of the day, month and year to give us additional information on our skills and what we are learning through our lifetime: see Part 2 of this book for further information.

RED personality

Life goal: self-awareness / **Life gift**: courage

General traits

People with a red personality exude intensity, which is characteristic of this colour – a red personality's aura is bigger than life. Their presence in a room does not pass unnoticed – they make sure that they will attract attention by talking about themselves or by making strong, opinionated statements that cause sparkles.

Most of the time they wear clothes that are out of the ordinary, which can be either very flamboyant or ultra-conservative, aiming to make a statement with their appearance.

Reds can be self-disciplined, conscientious and discerning people of great integrity. They fight for truth and justice, with no sense of superiority. They are fiercely faithful to their principles, taking a loner's stance against society if necessary. Armed with plenty of courage, passion and fearlessness, reds can act as pioneers, revolutionaries, leaders of the troops. They want to do what is right; they are lovers of truth and justice.

Reds are deeply connected to their roots: they need to be aware of their family's history and support. Despite insular tendencies, they are aware of other people's emotions and needs, which makes them loyal and totally trustworthy friends. They are straightforward, sometimes so much so that they might come across as crude. They definitely have both feet on the ground.

Red personalities are thrifty with their money, and have mostly conservative views.

Red is related to the number 1, and therefore they like to look after themselves, sometimes becoming quite selfish. They live in the moment, and, if things are not going their way, they can easily explode, fume, shout and yell, shattering everything and everybody around them in the process. They seem to be 'in your face' until they achieve whatever they desire. Once this red fiery energy has been expressed, reds become calm and sympathetic as if nothing had happened just minutes ago. Because this fiery explosion consumes all their negativity, red personalities do not hold grudges.

Reds have a competitive spirit and a determined and decisive mind: they want to take over, to invent better situations; their will to succeed is as big as their fear of failure. We can find red personalities in top jobs, successfully handling the most challenging situations. Their achievements are remarkable, and their dedication to humanity's higher good is passionate; with great courage they are prepared to give their lives for what they believe is right.

When changes occur, reds are fantastic at adapting to them: onwards and upwards is their motto! From a young age they are constantly engaged in something that will challenge their physicality, leading groups, being hot headed and opinionated.

Tricky traits

Red is the colour of intensity and passion, which can lead to the corresponding personality being constantly impatient, expressing themselves with a fiery burst of ill temper, followed by serenity until the next outburst of anger. Good or bad, the feelings of reds are very intense. If this underlying anger is not expressed, it becomes a smouldering resentment towards themselves, other people and life in general. Then, reds feel cut off and alone.

To make up for this lack of companionship, reds can become full of self-importance, believing they cannot do anything wrong and that everyone – except for them – is 'bad'.

This resentful attitude towards life is also directly related to the red personality's resistance to accepting reality. Their anger leads to chronic dissatisfaction with themselves and their situation. It makes reds feel that life is not as it ought to be. Reds do not generally see themselves as angry but instead as 'under control', as always striving to do what is right.

When red personalities are in their lower self, they can be destructive, pushy, angry, rebellious, domineering, resentful, arrogant, self-righteous and defiant. They will trample on others' toes to advance. When they are insecure, shame and guilt will overcome them.

Health and well-being

Red personalities need great physical energy so that they can achieve what they think they deserve and wish for. Any kind of physical exercise – as challenging as possible – is a must for them, to burn off excess energy. Competitive games are recommended for reds, because striving to win is part of their nature. Correct deep breathing is fundamental to their well-being.

The colour red corresponds to the head and lungs. With many red personalities there is often an inferiority complex, and illness can too often result from not achieving their aims.

In the bedroom

Reds are born romantics and love very deeply with intense passion. They seek the security of a long-term relationship, as they like to feel part of a family unit. They sometimes surround themselves with unnecessary objects, their need for the excitement of acquisition overpowering them. Their bedrooms tend to have bright, vivid colours, bespoke pieces of furniture, *objets d'art* and sensual scents.

Their love-making is passionate and insatiable, patience not being reds' strongest trait; they are quite direct about an instant need for sex. A physically fit partner is recommended for them!

But red personalities can also be quite straight-laced, uncomfortable with nakedness, and are unlikely to spend much time dwelling on the *Kama Sutra*! A 'quickie' is often enough to satisfy a red's need to release their fiery energy.

However, reds are often adventurous and experimental, easily bored with the same routine; they will take the initiative and give everything they have during their union with a partner. Reds live intense lives.

It is advisable for reds to choose a partner with plenty of physical energy and practical ways of thinking. Personalities who are too generous are at risk of being exploited by reds.

In the family

Red personalities rule in their household: for example, they expect everybody to behave according to the red ideals – justice, courage, self-discipline, passion, thriftiness, wisdom.

Reds will create a highly protected environment for their family, keeping members away from nasty influences. Children of red parents are disciplined, law-abiding and idealistic. When reds are not balanced as parents, these admirable and highly principled people can become controlling, full of 'musts' and 'shoulds', always trying to improve everyone by moralising and lecturing.

Overacting to minor mistakes as if they were mortal sins and being arrogant and self-righteous are additional behavioural patterns that can be very intimidating. Reds often find it difficult to hug children, as they are barely aware of their own tender feelings.

Red children are full of physical energy, and need rules and a structured environment to adhere to. Knowing the family tree reassures them of their heritage and provides them with safety and security.

At work

A 'healthy' red personality is perfect for any leading position: highly principled, structured, ready to fight in order to achieve what they believe in, they will keep all employees working like clockwork!

Reds appreciate hard workers, and most enjoy befriending successful people. They prefer to work within a set of firm guidelines in an orderly, precise manner. They are predictable, with very little room for creativity or personal preferences.

Being busy is important for reds, and they like to have various challenges on the go. These should be short tasks that have structured outcomes, and reds need to be shown exactly how to do these tasks before starting on them, so that they know precisely what to do.

As reds are very direct, if someone annoys them, a sharp response may be directed at the individual concerned. Their resentment will not hang around for long, so ensure that the matter is cleared up quickly.

Reds will be motivated by telling them how well they are doing; a pat on the back will overcome many negative obstacles.

How best to handle reds

Red personalities need to be able to express their 'bad' emotions to others yet still be reassured that they are loved for who they are. It is a good idea to rate situations from 1 to 10, with 10 being catastrophic. Being imperfect does not turn them into monsters; on the contrary, it makes people respond to them with greater warmth.

The directness of reds is not meant to harm: it is part of their way of expressing themselves. Don't take what is said to heart – they really do not mean to hurt, and will soon forget their words. Remember that reds do not hold onto resentment: 'least said, soonest mended'.

Helpful hints when things get tough

Reds have strong physical and emotional energy, more than any other colour personality. They need to find positive and creative outlets for their energy: it extremely difficult for them to relax, and without releasing this energy there is a risk of exhaustion.

Pacing themselves is important, as reds tend to give everything to each new project they undertake, and as soon as they finish they have the need to hunt for another. To win at any cost can have consequences for their health, as they tend to keep their more delicate feelings to themselves. It is beneficial for reds to express kindness to other people and an interest in their feelings, and to share with them life's ups and downs.

Red affirmation

I accept all there is with gratitude

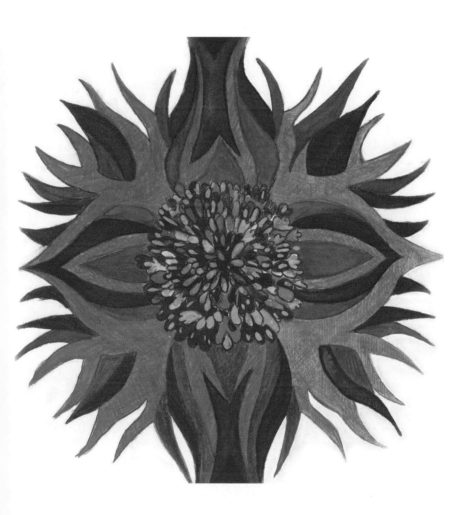

ORANGE personality

Life goal: self-respect / **Life gift**: creativity

General traits

People with orange personalities are warm, friendly, agreeable and quite easy-going, but they can also be very flamboyant due to the dynamic nature of this colour. Oranges are more assertive than aggressive, and an outrageous sense of humour is often a strong personality trait.

Oranges' greatest desire is to be important to others, to love and protect them, to be needed and appreciated, and to be physically close. They are the kind of highly emotional people who will notice the 'poor soul' sitting on their own at a party and take it upon themselves to cheer them up.

Oranges loves to socialise, so they are great at organising events and social gatherings with family and friends; they are team builders. Family is very important to them. They enjoy seeing interaction and also interacting themselves. Oranges can be heard as well as seen, with their loud dress sense and strong voices.

Deeply emotional, oranges can hide their vulnerable side by using humour and fun to protect themselves from any hurt or emotional discomfort. Oranges have to deal with issues of self-respect. They like nothing more than being appreciated by those they love.

Orange personalities have a tendency to 'let go' of issues quite quickly once they recognise the solutions and how best to incorporate them into their everyday world. They are very adaptable.

As orange is the colour of freedom, the corresponding personality does not like to be tied down to people, places or working environments. Oranges like to be flexible with their timings and to choose what to do and where on the spur of the moment.

Oranges can be very creative, and bring projects to life, as the colour orange relates to the sacral area of the body, which is associated with birthing. Unfortunately, completing a project can sometimes be more difficult. They have stamina and energy, and expect other people to match their energy levels.

When it comes to food, oranges love all kinds: food can be fairly dominant in their lives. Good food, good wine and good company is generally the orange's mantra! Food can therefore have a negative as well as positive effect on oranges, as it is not surprising that they are prone to weight gain and find dieting the hardest thing ever!

As adventurers, oranges need to be outside doing all sorts of things – camping, walking, skydiving, driving fast motorbikes. They are daredevils, and enjoy the adrenalin rush of dangerous sports. Many world explorers are orange personalities.

Oranges are great depression lifters, so if you are feeling a little down or want some support, then hunt out an orange. They are tactile individuals and are very fond of hugs and touching, which they enjoy immensely. But they are very capable of shutting off from affection if they feel that they have been hurt or that someone is being disrespectful to them.

Oranges are people's people: whatever they do is connected with relationships – unlike reds, who are always doing things for an impersonal principle. Oranges have open arms and open hearts to take in the whole world and bring comfort. They are the most caring of all the colour personalities.

Orange personalities are not competitive: *au contraire*, they are delighted with other people's success and leadership. They are supportive, bringing out the best in others – a very desirable trait for parents and teachers.

Oranges are also very good mediators and negotiators because they are able to see both sides of the coin. They feel secure and empathetic; they are warm and humble people who make the world a better place with their unconditional love and kindness.

Tricky traits

Oranges can become lazy, and tend then not to get things done. Sometimes this overindulgent attitude can lead to arrogance, especially in orange children, who expect to get everything they want without putting in any effort.

Oranges can also become lazy about their appearance and health, and if they are not careful they can 'let go' of themselves, and have to deal with the outcome later. Attention to preventative health measures is important – visiting the dentist, doctor, chiropodist, etc. – for oranges to be in 'tip-top' condition; their eating habits need to be watched. Comfort eating is natural for an emotional orange.

Issues of self-respect, especially in relationships, can be the cause of several illnesses based on the lower abdomen, such as lower back pain, IBS and period irregularities.

If oranges find themselves in a fearful situation, they can physically feel it in their gut. They can become unpredictable, indecisive and domineering, patience goes out the window, and everyone around them is told what to do and made to feel guilty. When oranges become seriously unbalanced they can become aloof, egotistical, self-centred and uncaring; they also suffer all kinds of psychosomatic illnesses – a response to the need for attention. Jokes can turn spiteful when resentment creeps in, and lack of patience becomes more acute.

Health and well-being

Oranges love risk, so their health may suffer if they put their body under strain by jumping out of planes, hurling themselves off bridges or driving very fast cars or motorbikes. They are also very sensitive to noise, negative and direct energies, and hard conditions, as they use their 'gut' feeling as a guide for life.

As oranges also like abundance, they are prone to overindulge with food and drink, so they can be susceptible to gaining weight. They are also emotional, and may use food as an antidote to dealing with negative emotions. Diet is very important to oranges for maintaining good health, and periods of relaxation are very helpful to rebuild an orange's energy.

This emotional nature when suppressed can create physical issues for oranges, but can be addressed by incorporating creative and interesting pursuits into everyday life. Anything that is not manifested through fun and creation for oranges will have a negative effect on their psyche, leading to laziness and self-absorption.

To make an orange feel healthy and well, tell them how important and helpful they are in your life; also, that you would not be where you are without their loving help. This can bring instant recovery!

In the bedroom

Oranges are very emotional, and will look for a partner in the bedroom who is not just passionate but also expresses feelings. Looking to the adventurous side of oranges, the bedroom is a great place to experiment, but oranges do need to make sure they are sincere in their love-making. As tactile individuals, hugs and kisses throughout the day are important to oranges: these can be as exciting to them as the actual sexual act.

Self-respect is the orange personality's core ideal, and this is also important in the bedroom. Sex – and lots of it – is good for oranges, because they have untiring, hot-hot-hot energy, but they must not feel that they are doing it for the sake of someone else's happiness or ends.

The more apricot shades of colour (orange mixed with white) are great when used in the bedroom to encourage fun, humour and communication. Food can also play an important role here, and a bedroom picnic would be an added bonus to orange lovers. Make it sweet and sour to cover all bases. Also, why not add some soft music for ambience? Oranges love to move to music!

The colour orange is associated with the sacral chakra and the sexual organs, so sexual pleasure is important to oranges to help with their overall well-being and self-respect. Keep oranges emotionally happy, and they will enjoy love-making; upset them and there will be no love-making (no food either!).

In the family

The orange personality as a parent can be great fun and creative, using their energy to connect with their children easily. As oranges have a huge amount of energy, they are great at helping to develop sporting talents in their children as well as creative pursuits. Oranges work well in groups of family members and also in family get-togethers and social situations.

Sometimes, oranges find it hard to apply discipline and structure, unlike the other colours, and with a tendency to be children themselves they can become too 'matey' with the kids and fail to take an authoritative role.

Oranges like to travel, so the family may have a caravan or motor home so they can just up and take a holiday whenever they are able.

Being stationary all the time is not easy for orange parents: house moves may occur quite often.

Orange children have a great sense of humour. They like to be extrovert – possibly budding actors or dancers – and show everyone what they are up to. Clowning around is a very orange thing. This may cover up a more sensitive side to their personality, so be aware that humour can sometimes hide pain.

Orange children will be creative, and love to make things from nothing – make sure you have enough space to exhibit their masterpieces.

However, orange children can become lazy if they lose interest, and when they become teenagers the bedroom becomes one of their favourite places. But, most of the time, orange children are a delight to have around!

At work

When it comes to the working environment, oranges need to be doing lots of creative tasks and also be free with their time. Many oranges are self-employed and in the creative arts, allowing freedom of expression at all levels. Oranges are photographers, artists, dancers, sculptors.

Oranges also love to travel, be that physically or mentally, and like to experience cultures and foods of any kind.

Many sports people are orange personalities because they have the energy of this warm colour and they also like the attention that these occupations can bring. Rally drivers and people seeking adventure in a work situation also tend to be oranges.

Oranges also like to be with as many other people as possible, so the social and teaching professions will attract oranges. Usually you will find them organising the social club or social outings for the organisation.

Oranges like to give birth to new ideas, although sometimes they can find it difficult to stay with the project all the way to its end. They need to have good discipline to see a job through.

Working with an orange means giving them varied tasks and deadlines – which you will need to check frequently to see how they are progressing – otherwise, if they are bored, they will become distracted and take an interest in something else.

Oranges are those people who will make cups of tea at work for colleagues and who will jump up to give a comforting hug to a workmate that has a hard day.

Oranges like their freedom, so you may find that they are self-employed with no boss, as this gives them flexibility. They can also spread themselves widely, with lots of ideas and projects on the go.

How best to handle oranges

Give oranges freedom to express their creativity and also make sure that you keep track of any deadlines they have so that they do not fall too far behind. Oranges hide their hurt and disappointment with humour and jokes: do look out for overzealous humour, as this usually hides something quite painful.

Oranges can be arrogant, thinking they know it all and wanting to help as many people as possible. If they are being overbearing, make them aware of this clearly and gently – cutting them down is not helpful, as they are very emotional.

The best thing you can do for an orange is to allow them to be genuinely helpful.

When wooing an orange, play to the emotions – romantic gestures are taken to heart and can heal any past upset quickly. Oranges do not hold onto negative emotions for long – they are very optimistic and fun when well balanced.

As friends, oranges like to have a busy social life and love to chat and invite people around to eat – a favourite pastime. Most oranges we know are great cooks! So, take them up on their invitations – their evenings will be lively and sociable!

Helpful hints when things get tough

For oranges, when things get tough they need to throw themselves into dancing, singing and creative pursuits. Their ability to 'let go' will come to the fore, and they can balance their deep emotions with feeling free.

Oranges' talent for 'daredevil' antics can lead them into doing something that could be dangerous when they are not in the right space.

If an orange is feeling resentful, perhaps expressed as 'I am dying and it's your fault for hurting me' or 'Without me you would never have managed', then they need to let go of loving other people with expectations of gratitude from them; instead, they need to learn to use their warm and caring nature to love themselves without thanks or repayment from others.

Orange affirmation

I am free, happy and creative. I open my eyes to abundance and I let go of anything that is no longer of benefit to me

YELLOW personality

Life goal: self-esteem / **Life gift**: clarity

General traits

Happy and cheerful, yellow personalities are great to have around at a social gathering. They are gifted with creativity, imagination, artistic talents, versatility and a good nature. Their enthusiasm is contagious. They are here to make the most of themselves. Chatting with people on a wide range of subjects from cookery to politics, yellows have the ability to use their mental strength to be knowledgeable about almost everything.

Yellows are a blessing to have around, and excellent at giving hope to others who might be feeling down. For them, success means really enjoying what they doing – whatever that might be. They remind people that life is a pleasure, to be approached positively. Of all the colour personalities, yellows are the most childlike – full of healthy curiosity and playfulness. They are authentic, modest and genuine.

Books, magazines, gadgets, technology, games and puzzles have a magnetic effect on yellows, stimulating their curious brains. With a healthy dose of competitive spirit plus their many talents, they are rarely upstaged. Yellows are here to be a success, to be stars and to make an impression!

Yellows find people fascinating, and effortlessly become friendly with others: they are great networkers. The ability to write is also prominent – interviewing and research are key areas of careers for yellows. They are good at getting information out of people.

In a more personal space they like to be involved with like-minded people: they would rather choose a small group of 'interesting' individuals over a larger gathering. Generous at all levels – material, emotional and spiritual – they need to be careful not to be overgenerous or wasteful.

At times, it is hard for a yellow to relinquish control over a project, and this can create some negativity. The trait of this personality to become somewhat stubborn and destructive may be quite apparent. Letting go of the outcome is one of the yellow personality's greatest challenges.

Relinquishing control may affect the self-esteem of yellows negatively – feelings of 'not being good' enough may appear: a common trait in yellow personalities.

Very often yellows can become ungrounded, as they tend to use all their mental energy and can become overwhelmed. This can lead to issues such as being unable to sleep due to an excess of mental activity and an increased need to over-analyse everything.

Dressing up in an assortment of clothes and having a wardrobe that contains all sorts of wonderful accessories appeals greatly to a yellow. This allows them to take on the different roles they so enjoy playing!

Yellows spend money as easily as they make it. They are capable of making rash decisions, spending any amount on anything from their career through to luxury holidays and house purchases. Because making money is so easy for them, sometimes they are not sympathetic to people who struggle financially – a yellow can't help but think, 'If they only applied themselves, they could earn a great living.'

Yellow personalities are highly sensitive: great receptors of people's energy, and they sense a situation before it is in the open. However, their identification with external energies can make them ill. They use logic to make sense of life: 'Black is black and white is white – why would anybody want to confuse these facts?' This logical approach acts as filter to their high sensitivity.

Tricky traits

Yellow personalities sometimes rush things rather than taking a steady pace, and bad results from quick decisions made by 'gut feel' rather than using logic can give rise to negative self-esteem.

When yellows are unable to share their positive yellow qualities with other people, they turn into self-centred egotistical creatures, feeling rejected and inadequate. They may then use others to get what they want.

If a yellow is out of balance, then their personality may become a little sour (like a lemon): when challenged, their words can be direct and biting. Their natural humour can become sarcastic and somewhat critical, although this is sometimes channelled at themselves. Self-criticism then becomes a very prominent problem to overcome.

Yellows have an ability to show the world only one side of their personality, which may conceal the truth about their circumstances. This makes them great actors, but can also allow them to lie to themselves about their situation. In the worst case, yellows can be pathological liars, arrogant, pretentious, superficial, sneaky, two faced and empty.

Health and well-being

Yellow personalities need to be gentle on themselves: their sensitive stomachs mean that food needs to be nutritious and digestible. A glass of warm water with lemon juice first thing in the morning is great for everyone, but additionally gives yellows the benefit of cleansing the liver and clearing any mucus and acid that their system has held onto overnight.

Yellows can experience problems with their liver, kidneys, pancreas and gallbladder, and need to help the body increase its ability to clear any toxins.

Yellow personalities are continuously on the go mentally, and can become ill when they reach exhaustion. Because they give a great deal of energy to others, they must take time to regroup and repair. Meditation or chi gung will balance a yellow's overactive mind.

In the bedroom

Yellow personalities have a light-hearted and energetic approach to sex. They are happy to experiment, but it has to be with someone they trust. Yellows are charming yet unpredictable: because of this they make exciting lovers (but also capable of trading in and trading up if a partner is too boring or possessive).

Yellows like lots of new ideas in the bedroom, and can become easily bored by the same old routine. Dressing up in all sorts of disguises suits the yellow personality, acting out different scenarios to excite both parties. Erotic literature stimulates their active brain and triggers new ideas for love-making. Although alcohol can make us all more relaxed, it can unleash abandonment in the bedroom and make yellows interesting and excellent sexual partners.

For some yellows, a choice of sexual partners may not be unusual, as this offers exciting times in the bedroom.

If self-esteem is lacking, then a yellow may be conscious of how they look in the bedroom, and therefore will need to build up trust with their partner to achieve a fulfilling sex life. They may also fall for the 'wrong' people – those who offer emotional relationships but are really interested only in sex.

A neat and tidy bedroom, elegantly decorated, will make a yellow feel totally at home. Good lighting is also very important for them, because light is so much of their core personality.

In the family

Yellow personalities as mothers and fathers encourage their children to learn as much as they can from books and education. Male and female parents are both fairly independent – and they like their children to become equally so by instilling the value of independence early in their lives.

When negativity becomes part of parenting or there is too much drama in a parent's life, there is a risk that the yellow parent will want to control their children and find it hard to let go. If a child does not behave as a parent expects, then there may be harsh words or bitter discussions where things get said that may never be rectified.

It is important that parents encourage positive self-esteem from an early age in a yellow child. This will benefit the child in the long run, and although encouragement to achieve academically is required, it is not possible to push a yellow child until they are ready. Yellow personalities may achieve better academically as they grow older and study later in life, when self-esteem is higher.

Creativity and play, drama schools and game clubs are excellent tools for the yellow child, and, if they excel in any one of these areas, then it is important for the parent to encourage their child's ability.

At work

In the workplace you will find project managers to be yellows – efficient and organised. System processes and clear and precise instructions can be created by yellow personalities. They are also excellent at coming up with new ideas and seeing 'the bigger picture' to create overall concepts, which others can bring into reality.

With their inquisitive minds and their natural ability to analyse, yellow personalities can make excellent scientists.

Yellow personalities are great networkers. The ability to write is also prominent, and interviewing and research are key areas of careers for yellows. They are good at getting information out of people and translating this for magazines, books, etc.

Yellows light up the workplace with their style, charm and high spirits. They are polished, popular and focused on success not feelings.

How best to handle yellows

Yellows need encouragement to help boost their self-esteem. When they are being defensive it is possible that they will communicate directly – which can be quite blunt and sharp. Your reaction is important, so if you wish to get the best out of a yellow, don't challenge them directly but instead remember that they are hiding a lack of self-esteem as they project a happy, sunny image all of the time – underneath, they are feeling vulnerable. Approach the issue at a later date so that you can discuss it openly.

Allow yellows to help you problem solve any issue using their analytical mind, and thank them for it as well. Always be meticulously clear to a yellow about how you feel, and don't be at all sentimental. Do be careful when dealing with happy, sunny personalities: sometimes they are able to use this to deceive you into a false sense of security and then take what they need.

Yellows love words, so when you want to surprise them and tell them how wonderful it is when their sunny disposition and happy personality lights up your world, choose a poem, card or plaque to express how you feel.

As yellows love being in control of nearly everything, make sure that you have your own space and that when you need to do anything, be clear and direct in your intentions. Also remember that they are in their minds a great deal of the time, which can make them ungrounded – help them to do activities instead of thinking about activities.

Helpful hints when things get tough

Yellows need to be doing something physical to ground themselves in the everyday and not lose themselves in their minds. Massages, meditation, swimming and health spa days are excellent at relaxing and re-energising a yellow person.

When life becomes challenging, it is necessary for yellows to stop their constant analysis and instead allow things to develop. This can only be achieved by remembering that they are part of a bigger picture and that things will happen at the right time. A few deep breaths at moments of overactive thinking will help to bring a yellow back to their body.

Yellow affirmation

I am clear that life has my best interests at heart and I let go
of any control

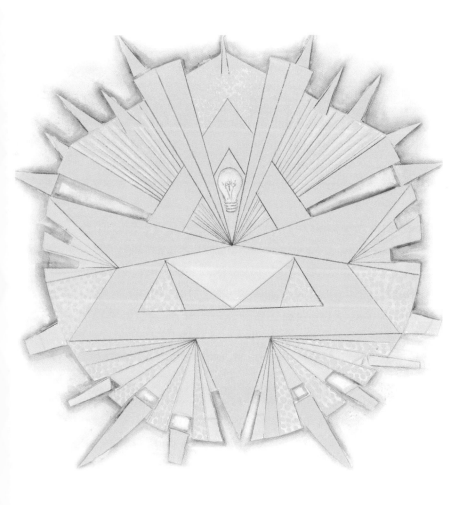

GREEN personality

Life goal: self-love / **Life gift**: harmony

General traits

Greens like to have balance, harmony and stability in all aspects of their lives. They are practical, down to earth and at their happiest when they are amongst nature. Their ambition is to become self-actualised, and because they are so close to their hearts they strive to give meaning to pain.

Practical greens are great to have around in a crisis, as they tend to be calm, and can take control of any situation. They are dependable, stable and in harmony with the world and their environment. They are kind, generous, compassionate and great listeners, so can become faithful and loyal friends. Anyone who crosses the path of a green is richer for the experience, because this hard-working, faithful personality has a balancing and steadying effect on others.

Learning and gaining knowledge in all sorts of subjects interests greens, as they are intelligent and have a knack for understanding new concepts and ideas very quickly. Reading all sorts of literature, watching varied television programmes and taking an interest in those around them gives them the ability to see both sides of any situation, and they may well take a role as a peacemaker or mediator.

Greens like to feel that they are good citizens and part of the local or wider community. They have high moral standards – doing the right thing is very import to a green.

Greens like to 'belong', whether to a group or to an individual or family. They need to be accepted, admired and appreciated for all the good that they do for a community as well as for their family and friends.

They make great hosts and hostesses, making sure everyone is well fed and watered. They enjoy organising events, and have the ability to communicate the right information at the right time. Social skills are instinctive to greens, so they are fabulous to have around when starting up a new group, business or community idea.

As true observers, greens enjoy letting the world go by and watching it from the best positions, like a café. The colour green relates to the heart: when green personalities are truly appreciated for their support and practical approach to helping others, they feel comfortable with themselves.

The quick mind of a green and their understanding of the human perspective are key to this personality. Greens are able to appear innocent and seemingly know nothing about the world, but they are great readers of people, and often keep that psychic ability to themselves.

Greens love to accumulate things, but these are usually of high quality. This bodes well for a business venture: greens are great with purchasing and the plan, but find it much harder to execute the necessary tasks. If they delegate well, then they can create profitable and successful businesses. Behind multimillion-pound companies there is often a green personality, manifesting their dream.

Greens wear their hearts on their sleeves. They love talking about their feelings for hours on end; by airing their thoughts to a listening ear, they are better able to understand themselves.

The colour green represents growth and new beginnings. Green personalities therefore tend to stay young in body and mind, as they continually grow and transform due to their need to be in balance with life.

Tricky traits

Greens need to take responsibility for their own lives and situations, and blaming others is common for unbalanced greens. Unfortunately, blaming doesn't accomplish anything apart from keeping them stuck and dis-empowered. This can lead to envy and jealousies, always wanting what other people have: they become 'the green-eyed monster'.

Greens love to gossip – it is a sign of their need to belong, and although it might seem harmless chatter, negative gossip can be dangerous and destructive in the wrong hands.

Greens also need to appreciate what they've learned and already accomplished. They are typically perfectionists, fearing that nothing is ever good enough. Greens can neglect their own needs and spend too much time caring for others. They then become disappointed and resentful. Greens need to make sure that they don't become too self-righteous and complacent.

Greens can suffer from self-hatred, self-destructive behaviour and excruciating self-consciousness. They can feel isolated, desperate and melancholic, unable to find comfort anywhere or from anybody.

Health and well-being

Greens love their food, and some greens can find it hard to lose weight. As this colour affects the stomach, the upper right side of the body and the right arm, it is important that they do not overdo rich food, as this can lead to high blood pressure and being overweight.

Some greens may suffer from food allergies and intolerances. A balanced diet with gentle exercise is required for a green body to be in harmony. Greens can endure long periods of work pressure, but they need time to rebuild when they are suffering from lethargy and circulation problems.

The colour green also relates to the lungs and breathing. Greens may thus suffer early in life with breathing issues, asthma or chest conditions, but these soon disappear as they get older.

In the bedroom

As greens are all about love, the bedroom is the place for them to express this love – it is not just for sex. There needs to be equilibrium between the head and the heart for greens to enjoy sex, meaning that they have both a heartfelt need for their partner and a need for a connection on the mental level for sex to be fulfilling.

When a green falls in love it is not with great passion but is more gentle and steady. The need for balance in all aspects of life overrides the need for passion and action.

Preparation is the name of the game for a green – the lead up to the actual act is just as important as the act itself. Gentle flirtation using words, a text message or sexual innuendo will activate a green into thinking about how best to please their partner's needs.

Greens can be tactile and want to touch and feel – skin on skin is important when love-making. Gentleness, safety and compassion outweigh passion, so fast and furious sex tends to be uncomfortable for a green, especially if they have high moral standards and ethics.

Greens do however love to experiment with different positions and techniques, and they also require feedback on performance, sometimes during love-making and especially after. Tantric sex, the *Kama Sutra* and exotic fiction can be interesting for a green to experiment with, and telling a green how fantastic they are and how much they are loved keeps the bonds in the relationship extremely strong. If they feel insecure they can be extremely jealous in a relationship.

Green is an earthy colour, so fresh sheets and essences of pine, olive and grass can balance the equilibrium for a stressed green in the bedroom. Some greens can also appear naive sexually, but you may find that they really are quite streetwise and will try their hand at anything.

Sometimes sex for a green can actually mean love, so they can be rather demanding when it comes to how much sex they would like. They can also become possessive of people and use sex as a tool to manipulate relationships.

In the family

Green parents will usually have an active interest in community projects or perhaps Greenpeace or other worldwide charities that protect the environment.

Plenty of time will be spent outdoors doing sport or family activities, and it is quite likely that camping and caravanning holidays will be favourites on a green parent's list. They will be encouraging of their children in all aspects of their life, showing compassion and kindness when it is required.

Greens do like balance around the home, so arguments can make them overanxious and irritated, but they are happy to have their friends' children round to play, and will keep them fed and looked after until they go home. Sometimes they can be too accommodating, just to keep the peace.

Green children have quite a lot of friends, and enjoy socialising with all sorts of people including grown-ups and elderly members of the family. They observe what is going on around them and have a great ability to sense positive and negative situations.

At school they will pretty much 'fit in' with other children, but may be attracted to join a group that is not part of the 'in' crowd, to enable them to support and help others less able to adapt. They are usually quite bright, but can find school boring, as they are not necessarily interested in the everyday details of many lessons and are more interested in wider subjects such as religion, history or architecture.

Show them love and attention, and a green child will excel at anything that they put their mind to. But always talk positively and patiently, as they are easily hurt. They are social and generally happy children.

At work

Generous with money, greens like to earn it, and can be quite business orientated, so they tend to work for themselves Many successful entrepreneurs are greens, and this is also because they are very good at delegating the detail work, as they are not interested in doing it themselves.

Greens make excellent counsellors, social workers, psychologists and doctors, and they are great at listening and also have an exceptional talent at viewing others people's problems with empathy, clarity, respect and care.

As greens always fit into their environment socially and are good at communication, they will be adaptable and flexible in the workplace.

They can work successfully in the caring professions and help make exacting decisions about health and illnesses.

If greens trust their instincts, which come from the heart, they can be very successful and make a lot of money. Green is the colour of money in the Western world, and greens feel safe and balanced when they have enough money. They usually contribute to charities and projects that are close to their heart.

How best to handle greens

Give greens love, as it fulfils their main need to belong and feel safe and secure. A 'thank you' is sufficient for a green, and will allow them to extend further courtesies to you. Always lend a kind ear to a green.

Greens don't like to be told what to do, and are very strong willed, so requests to greens should be made in a balanced manner; let them think it was their idea. Remember that they have high moral standards, so don't ask them to do anything that could offend them.

Greens are stubborn when they don't get their way, and if they become over-possessive, selfish or miserly, remind them gently of their true nature – caring, compassionate, nurturing.

Helpful hints when things get tough

Try to get greens to go for a walk in the country – they will soon replenish their energies. Talk to them about positive things, maybe purchasing an interesting film or book for them on a subject they are drawn to, or take them to a concert or involve them in an environmental project.

Make a green smile with a joke or some humour to relax them, so they don't take life too seriously.

Being creative with their hands – doing crafts, gardening and DIY jobs – but also finding creative ways to solve those everyday little challenges will bring a green's passion to life. The results are usually very beautiful.

Green affirmation

My true nature is love. I constantly surround myself with balance and harmony

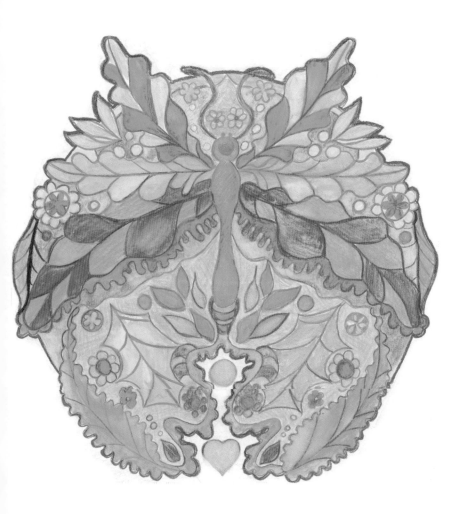

BLUE personality

Life goal: self-expression / **Life gift**: truth

General traits

The most characteristic trait of blue personalities is their great ability to communicate with anyone – whether they are talking to a king or a pauper, their obvious interest and ease is visibly apparent. Their eyes light up when they hear happy news, and they are very willing to 'lend an ear' when things are not so good.

Blue personalities have a natural ability to know what is right and what is wrong. They are clever, resourceful, adventurous and productive, and will 'have a go' at anything at least once, often trying again if the outcome was less than positive the first time around.

Blue as a colour cools and heals: these qualities relate very much to the personality's colour. Blues can seem detached when things become a little heated! They feel deeply, and struggle at times to show their tender side, which can make them appear a little remote.

A blue's life purpose is to help, comfort and support the less fortunate. They are very caring, and will make sure that their close circle is well looked after, sometimes to their own detriment; they live following the five virtues – truth, kindness, wisdom, justice and love. Blues have a great capacity for love, and they readily ask forgiveness when they do something wrong. With these qualities, they make sincere and loyal friends.

Blue is also the colour of trust, and blue personalities like to be able to trust someone before they create what can be a very deep or close friendship or relationship. If they are lied to they will sever any ties, and verbal exchanges can become direct and harsh, making the relationship unsalvageable. Clear communication is a positive keynote for blues and in dealing with this personality.

Intellect and knowledge are high on life's values for a blue: they love to learn, and have a constant thirst for information on all sorts of subjects. They are fascinated by words, whether heard or from reading, and they are very capable of expressing themselves through writing. They love to have a variety of interests, but like the familiar, and tend to do things their way even if there is a better way of doing something – making them a little inflexible and stubborn.

A blue's life's ambition is to know all there is there to know; they want to be rational, knowledgeable and wise; they thrive on studying. They are gifted with a high intellect, and can understand and explain things that the average person would never dream of. They are also excellent at reading people's body language and behaviour, 'sussing' them out in just a few minutes after their first encounter.

Sometimes blues can struggle to see other people's point of view, and tend to search for like-minded people to support their own beliefs and systems. They can also become susceptible to the 'fear of lack', which means that they can be tight with money or hoard items, worrying that there is not enough to go round.

Words and communication are closely connected to the blue personality, and their tone and quality of voice can have a calming effect on everyone around them. They make great orators, and when they have a passion for their subject and choose to communicate orally, they can be direct, deeply moving and persuasive. They are excellent at making complex, obscure information relevant to others.

When blues are insecure they can become very detached and shut away from life, so that they can protect themselves. This can sometimes be hard for a partner who has warmer colours and is more expressive, because they may feel inadequate and unable to fulfil the blue's wishes. But if blues learn to use their excellent communication skills well to explain their emotions, then balance will prevail.

Tricky traits

Blue personalities can be somewhat snobbish, eccentric, reclusive and cold, even to the extent of appearing frigid and spiteful. They can show an unforgiving and moody temperament, which may lead them to becoming 'stuck in rut'. They can also become nihilistic and pessimistic – feeling totally 'blue'.

Change is always difficult for blues. When feeling unsettled they can withdraw from the world and shut themselves away, hoping it will all go away – unfortunately, this rarely happens, and blues must confront issues whether they like it or not.

Blues love to hoard objects and knowledge, believing that if they let things go they will regret their loss and be unable to replace them; when insecure, they tend to be tight with money.

Untidiness and unpredictability can have a negative effect on blues, making them feel overwhelmed. This creates anxiety, which can lead to worry about anything and everything, resulting in a bout of self-pity and a syndrome of 'poor me', and then withdrawal from reality.

Blues can also be masters of manipulation, so as to get an easy ride. They can do this quite subtly – and it not uncommon for them to suddenly 'drop a bomb' and then walk away without discussion, leaving others to pick up the pieces.

Health and well-being

As blues spend so much time helping others, they may ignore their own needs, and they can therefore put a great deal of strain on their own bodies without even being aware of the damage they are doing.

When blues realise the seriousness of an illness they are suffering from, they are quick to find solutions, either by visiting a doctor or taking an alternative route, seeking out a professional in the correct field.

The colour blue corresponds to the liver, gall bladder, the left arm and the upper left side of the body. With many blue personalities, over-activity, restlessness, inner dissatisfaction and critical states of mind bring nervous tension – the bane of a blue's life. This upsets the whole physical co-ordination of the body.

Meditation as a daily practice and finding a quiet time are very beneficial for blues, to allow them to rebuild their energies and to give them peace and harmony. They don't like to have their feathers ruffled, and will manipulate things to achieve an easy life. Blues can be subject to accidents and physical hurts that entail long periods of convalescence.

In the bedroom

When a blue is in love with their partner, they try to demonstrate this love in the most sincere and open way. They will do anything to please, always ready to follow wishes and instructions. Their childlike openness and curiosity accepts new ideas trustfully, and bedroom antics with a hot personality will fire their passion and push them to places they would never dream of going on their own initiative.

Once blues have made a commitment to their partner, their ability to make a deep and meaningful connection grows. Sex then becomes harmonious and relaxed, but if they become insecure they may detach from sex as a form of manipulation and to protect their privacy.

Blues love looking after their partner's needs, and can fuss around them. Reading to blues from sensual books (soft porn) or looking at erotic pictures together will work for them, because they love to learn; but be careful as this pure and sensitive personality will shrink away from 'dark' or 'hard' pornography.

Blues love a peaceful and orderly bedroom, which allows them to relax – low lights, freshly washed sheets, a few books always on the side table, gentle music and nice scents – but if you wish to spice up a blue personality's performance, add some red, orange, peach or apricot to the bedroom, to stimulate arousal.

In the family

Blue parents tend to be very hard working in all sorts of ways, generally helping other people as well as the family. Many blue parents spend their life earning money for their family, only to find that they have given up on their own aspirations and needs for the sake of the family, and may then in later years become full of self-pity.

Blue parents can also be rather aloof and hold back from being involved in physical activities with their young children, but their ability to communicate knowledge and information can motivate a child in many other areas of their personality.

Blue children can seem more aloof than the warmer colour personalities, and is not uncommon to find them with their head in a book or playing computer games. Blue babies are the quiet ones!

Blue kids also like to observe before joining in, and only make friends with people they trust. They also have a high boredom threshold, so make sure that they have enough to learn and to keep them occupied. Stimulate them with music, singing and communication.

When blue children become insecure they may detach from their friends and family and spend much time alone. This can lead to these kids 'feeling blue' and out of touch with the joy and freedom of being a child. Sometimes, blue children take their responsibilities for life too early and too seriously – surround them with orange and yellow to reconnect them to the joys of childhood.

At work

You will find many blues working in the caring professions, perhaps in hospitals, at the doctors or in care homes. You can also find them in charity organisations, helping to support social and humanitarian issues. Their gentle healing energy and soothing voices have an immediate positive impact on patients. Blues think and feel deeply, but keep their drama contained and rarely express how they are feeling.

Blue personalities like roles that have structures and are routine based, so that they feel safe and can relax in a regular environment. They are calm and tend not to create a volatile atmosphere unless they wish to manipulate an outcome to their benefit – when they will throw a spanner into the works and observe from afar what takes place. In general, blues are trustworthy and have integrity.

Blues also love to collect things. If they are working for themselves and buying and selling, they need to make sure that they are able to sell the items and not keep them for their own collections.

Blues are very astute with their business partners and suppliers, as they need to trust people before they make decisions. Sometimes this means that they are best at running their own business, as they can be inflexible when working in partnerships.

How best to handle blues

Be straight when you need to tell blues something – being clear and precise is the best communication style with this personality. Blues are virtuous and innocent and want to communicate love, wisdom, justice, kindness and truth, so do ask them for their advice on any matter; they will then feel that they are connecting with you and helping.

Don't take it personally when a blue seems remote and uncaring: this is just their natural way of behaving to rebuild their energy. Blues like a quiet life, so keeping away from confrontation will enhance their ability to communicate constructively; otherwise, they tend to shut down and become unable to communicate. Too many dinner parties and social gatherings are tiresome for blues, who would much rather spend their time studying.

Blues need to trust people, which means that there is a need for clarity and understanding in their relationships. Blues are very loyal, so make sure you let them know how important they are in your life and how much you trust them.

Helpful hints when things get tough

Blues should use their detachment to release themselves from the grip of anxiety. They need to learn that objects are not important, and that they don't need to hoard in order to reassure themselves that there will always be enough. Once this attachment to material things is controlled, they can be the compassionate and forgiving healers, sharing their deep knowledge with others.

Blue affirmation

At any moment all my needs are met. There is always enough for everybody

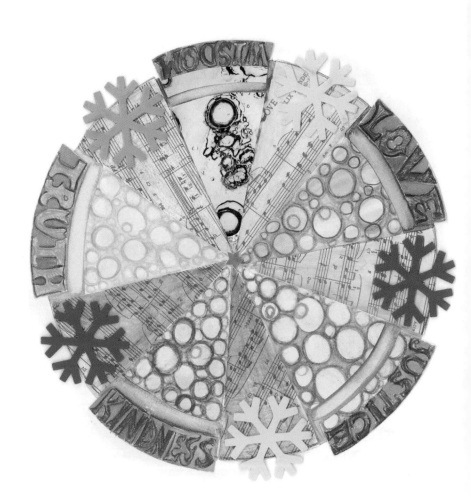

INDIGO personality

Life goal: self-responsibility / **Life gift**: intuition

General traits

Indigo personalities are fundamentally structured, organised and very independent. Indigos can be conscientious and hard-working, happily repeating the same tasks and duties day in and day out. Indigos feel safe with what they know, and are usually very good at what they do.

Justice, law and order are very important to indigos: they can be found involved in human rights movements when there are issues overseas or on the home turf. They identify with and fight for the disadvantaged. Their aim is to create stability and security in the world and in their personal circle.

Indigos can be creative, friendly and self-expressive. They are amusing, playful, childlike and endearing, which makes then very popular (even if they don't believe they are).

Indigos like receiving certification for the efforts they make, so they may sign up for many courses to underpin their already heightened intuitive knowledge. This gives them an air of authority. Indigos are also great to have around when there is a crisis because they respond in a cool and calm manner.

Sometimes this cool-colour personality can be seen as 'hard' or 'aloof' and unapproachable, but behind this exterior is a deep knowledge and understanding of the world around them.

Indigos are very conscious of and exceptionally good at whatever tasks they take on, but can overload themselves with chores. They need to learn to say 'no' and not wait until they resent the fact that everybody asks for their help.

The indigo personality may sometimes become moody and introspective: looking for higher truths in life they can become disillusioned, and this may lead to depression. They can also be indecisive because they strongly feel the division between the left and right sides of the brain. But they do have the ability to accept and balance the contradictory sides of themselves.

Indigos are loyal and good friends, always listening and not taking sides. They do not like confrontation, and prefer a balanced environment.

Indigos rely on intuition, and are able to see beyond the normal senses. Some indigos are therefore drawn to the psychic and clairvoyant world. This insight can be very useful in clearing problems or confused situations in life, and enables them to be excellent life coaches.

Indigo personalities are sensitive, courageous and idealistic. They excel in a happy and healthy family environment: home is important to them. They are unusually devoted to their family and friends.

Indigos cannot live life without a diary to plan events, and do not like surprises. If this organisation is not in place, then fear and anxiety can creep in and create much self-doubt, with the result that indigos become unable to take risks and expand their lives.

Indigos love rituals and traditions, and they will use much of the past to create their futures.

Tricky traits

The trickiest trait for an indigo is fear – of the unknown, of the future, of risks – which means that they may never achieve their goals as their fear is just too great. Indigos can then become judgemental and impractical. This can create a negative stubbornness to act, which may result in them feeling put upon and even martyred. When this negativity arises, indigos can create a drama out of nothing, so that the fear and anxiety they feel is shared around. This can lead to fanatical and obsessive behaviour at times.

Instead of seeking help, indigos will disconnect and hide away from conflict, which can increase their fear further. This may give rise to addiction – to pills, work or victimisation. If they seek help, they are the ones who are often 'in therapy' for years, endlessly seeking parent figures.

A negative indigo may exhibit intolerance and inconsiderate behaviour, making it hard for their family and friends to support and help them with the situation. This can result in the indigo becoming isolated, possibly leading to depression.

Health and well-being

Fear is one of the main issues that indigos need to conquer; and fear of ill health may be a major hurdle to overcome. Indigos are very cool blues, and it is not always possible to know how they are truly feeling because they keep much of themselves hidden.

Depression is a common problem for indigos as they can feel 'very blue'. Indigos also have an addictive trait, and some may find that they are addicted to work, alcohol, illness, religion or qualifications among many other things.

If addiction is present, it is very difficult habit for indigos to break, as they do not like to be told what to do and are very sensitive to how people perceive them. With perseverance and tapping into their intuitive side, they can find answers and bring balance into their lives.

Indigos are very sensitive, and allergies and chemical imbalances are quite common, and there may be problems with hormones, especially during the female life changes. The colour indigo is associated with the third eye, so there may also be problems with eyesight, cataracts, glaucoma and other sinus problems.

In the bedroom

For the indigo personality, the sexual act is more of a connection of souls rather than a physical connection. The intensity with which an indigo loves is very strong, and once you are their partner, you will be their partner for life.

Indigos are able to camouflage their personalities in the bedroom, sometimes seeming austere and authoritative, but sensitivity lurks beneath this surface, and once they know that they are not breaking any rules sexually and trust their partner completely, they can be dynamic lovers – especially if they believe that this match was divinely made. Their dreams and fantasies can be rather 'out of this world', and some indigos are happy to experiment with the more kinky side of sex, which may lead to addictive behaviour if they are not careful.

Indigo is the colour of midnight – the best time to play – and when an indigo's feminine energies are strong, they have rather fascinating fantasies. They like drama, and being an actress or actor in the bedroom does not seem alien to them once they have their partner's trust.

Indigo relates to the third eye, so indigos like fragrances in the bedroom to help stimulate the atmosphere, along with candles and items that imply that it is now dark and fun can begin. They are also turned on by visual stimuli – soft and even hard porn may be interesting to them. Their very own dungeon may not be off the menu for some indigos, though you would never know it from their everyday life!

In the family

Indigo parents can sometimes be hard to understand. There are usually fairly strict house rules, and when issues need to be addressed, indigo parents will be just. They are sincere in what they say and have great wisdom – which is sometimes offputting because they always seem to be right.

Sometimes, the rigid way that indigos do things does not allow space for new and creative ideas, so growth within an indigo family can take time. Stubbornness and narrow-minded views can cause friction, but, when balanced, the indigo parent can be loving and very practical.

Being drama queens and kings, life is never dull with an indigo parent, and they are always faithful to the family and in their closest relationships. They will have moments when things 'come out of the blue' and surprise you, but structure and organisation override random acts.

Indigo children are very sensitive to energy and emotions, although they may not show that they are. They are fascinated by new technologies, and are very intuitive. When they love a subject they will lap it up, but if it does not interest them they will switch off. They have wise, deep eyes, cannot tolerate lies, authoritarian rules or the unauthentic. ADHD and other learning disorders may be more common in indigo children than in other personalities. Be gentle with an indigo child; they are here to help us learn more about our changing planet.

At work

Indigos know best, and sometimes it is really hard to disagree with them. They can come across as cold and hard, but this is just self-protection, and at times they will let their guard down with people that they trust.

Indigo personalities like structure, so projects need deadlines, and tasks need to be done in a certain order. Once a framework is in place, it is hard for indigos to change it, as they will believe that it is the best way of dealing with the task.

Indigos are honest and hold integrity in high regard, so you can trust them with money and confidential information. They have a tendency not to talk about private matters unless they believe that it would be detrimental to the workplace if facts are not brought to light.

If working at a crisis centre or in an environment where crises occur frequently, indigos are good to have around. They calm down the atmosphere and use their organisational ability to follow through a process. They can be excellent teachers with high ideals.

Indigos will always defend others' rights and believe in the truth: they will take a fall to see that justice is done.

How best to handle indigos

It is important to understand that indigos are highly sensitive. They will feel your tension, anxiety or anger, and this will affect them physically or mentally. In relationships, trust is the most important thing to them; they are completely monogamous, and need you to be the same. You have to be able to allow an indigo to be who they are: if you try to remake them, you will create depression and resistance that will cause them to pull away – and you won't get them back. They will be faithful to you as a partner or friend, but they definitely need their space, so do not crowd them.

You may find indigos' know-it-all attitude annoying at times, but they do have a connection with a higher source that most personalities would be envious of, if only they could understand it. Their keenness to analyse their dreams may seem trivial to you, but for them it is an important process that helps them to progress: be supportive. If an indigo offers you advice, listen carefully: it may not seem right at the time, but somewhere down the track you will find that they were correct – they have uncanny foresight.

Helpful hints when things get tough

Indigos need to remind themselves of the cosmic and profound wisdom of the universe by looking for positive daily actions such as prayer or meditation. They should introduce a positive ritual into their day, such as a small shrine with bright colours and positive messages, so they can feel that they are connected.

Friends of an indigo need to be careful to spend enough time with them so that they do not feel alone and isolated. If addiction is an issue, then maybe find them some help through counselling – but be careful how you approach this as they may be offended.

Indigo affirmation

I am responsible for all my actions and I use faith to guide me

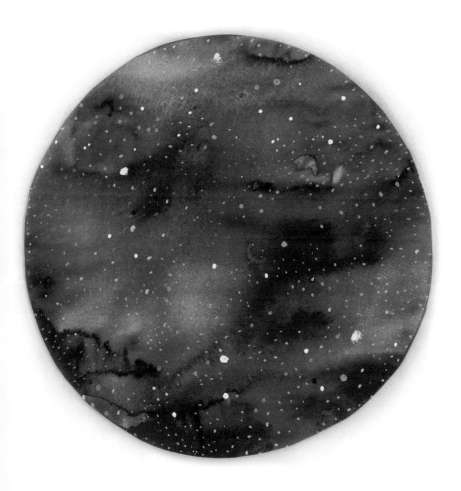

VIOLET personality

Life goal: self-knowledge / **Life gift**: inspiration

General traits

Violet personalities are intellectual, philosophical, imaginative, solitary and physically gifted. They are extremely strong personalities. They are private, although not necessarily unapproachable. They are here to understand that every living thing is sacred, and they have aspirations to bring the human race to a new phase of abundance and perfection. Their mission is to serve 'the highest' with joy.

They are blessed with good physical, intellectual and spiritual strength. These qualities are necessary for them to make the changes they desire in their lives as well as in the lives of others.

Violets are those individuals who know how to enjoy life to the full, thriving with every new and pleasurable experience. They enjoy pampering themselves; they don't usually suffer from existentialistic angst, self-hatred or doubt. They seem to be forever young, truly happy just being alive.

This personality is finely tuned to the higher vibrations, which opens the violet's sensitivity to artistic pursuits. They can create the most magnificent masterpieces or write the most inspirational poetry or music, as much of their inspiration is channelled from a higher source. They are highly disciplined in order to develop their talents.

Violets are psychic beings, and the solitude they seek intensifies this quality. They need a tranquil environment in which to live and work. They are in tune with nature, and avoid unauthentic things. They love to explore different myths and religions, and they will travel to places where they can learn more from them.

All the knowledge that violets accumulate needs to be shared with others; if not, violets can isolate themselves from society and become solitary. Some senior corporate managers are violets, using their inspiration to create unique organisations, because of their sensitivity, their aspiration for abundance and their natural connection to the higher vibrations.

Healthy violets are grateful for everything they have. Life for them is a gift full of wonders and joy. They are good, dignified leaders, often doing a lot for society. They have the gift of looking at things objectively and of being able to give practical advice. They love to be in motion, sometimes just for the sake of being active. They are exuberant, enthusiastic, energetic and optimistic. Violets often have connections with celebrities in political, artistic and intellectual fields, usually getting to know them through unusual circumstances.

Violets are lovely companions at dinner parties and social gatherings, and they always seem to have plenty of interesting things to talk about. Their charm leaves a lasting impression. Surrounded by beautiful, elegant, precious things and with their innovative minds, they contribute to the world with their generosity and style.

Violet personalities are usually self-confident and successful, but when they are not in their best state, they become critical of their behaviour, trying to find mistakes in everything they do and feeling bad for not being good enough. They might seem remote and cold, but this is camouflage for a very delicate soul that can easily get hurt.

Some violets feel that they have a sacred purpose in life, and are afraid that they might miss it if they are not in the right place or at the right time. This makes them eager for new experiences, filling up all their time and trying to keep their options open. As long as they are waiting for the magic to begin they are missing the magic that is happening here, right now.

Tricky traits

A violet's negative traits are impracticality, secretiveness, inapproachability, moodiness and laziness. They can also be unrealistic, creating a world of their own, so they need to be extra-careful not to cut themselves off from society.

From time to time, violets feel that they really don't want to be here on earth, and turn their colour in on themselves, which can create very negative patterns and thoughts.

Especially negative violet personalities are tragically snobbish and self-centred; nobody can trust them. They can betray and lie in order to achieve their purpose.

Violets can become hypochondriacs, finding imaginative diseases just to get attention. Their self-interest does not allow them to care about anybody else. They become introvert and they think they are the best and the greatest. Their intuitive qualities change into arrogance, and they use their metaphysical abilities to control everybody around them. If violets lose their scruples, nothing can stop them from achieving their evil goals; when this occurs, they can become extremely destructive.

When violets feel empty inside, they will hunt for 'good experiences' and a quick fix: they will avidly collect good experiences to fill this void – an obsession with food being a good example. They can become unrealistic, mixing up their needs with their wants: in constantly searching for reassurance they can end up feeling emptier and emptier.

Health and well-being

Violets need to have absolute faith that they are on the right path, so that they can follow their dreams and aspirations with all of their heart. They need to be aware of their tendency to self-criticism and, sometimes, of being perfectionist.

If you know a violet, a pat on the shoulder will encourage and reassure them. Remind them that they are here to serve a higher purpose.

Violets need to make time for meditation and prayer; once they feel confident that they are doing what they are here for, all their inner stress will be released, and their life will become more enjoyable.

The colour violet corresponds to the spleen, white blood cells and the sympathetic nervous system. Violets need to be selective regarding diet, as they can confuse need with want, and periods of relaxation are also necessary, to escape from too much social life.

Repression of emotions and feelings can result in poor physical health. The lower left side of the body and the left leg are often affected.

In the bedroom

Violets are sensitive and delicate: approach them with fine manners, a clean, well-groomed appearance and a little unconventionality; they love creative people.

Speak to violets straight to their hearts about the latest charitable activities around the world as well as your personal positive views that the world can be saved through 'sisterhood and brotherhood, love and understanding'.

Take violets to a large, sophisticated restaurant serving delicious food. Space is important to them as they can get a bit claustrophobic in small, untidy rooms, so a luxury hotel room will break any ice that might still be there after the fine meal.

Be knowledgeable about many subjects, as violets know a lot, and you don't want to bore them.

In return, violets will look after you and make sure that all your senses are 100% satisfied – violets don't do things halfway. They are born hedonists!

Acknowledge a violet's exquisite performance, and they will not only reward you with another union full of sparks but also with a generous gift next time they see you.

If you allow violets to have their space, they will keep on inviting you into their sanctuary. Remember to always go for the authentic – imitations or the artificial are a no-no if you want a violet's devotion. If you do win their devotion, a wonderful and generous life is ahead of you – sharing sweet times with your sumptuous violet while planning on saving the world together!

In the family

Violet personalities are generous, and they will happily spend all their money to buy the best for their families. They will choose the best schools, leisure activities, clothes and toys for their children, but in return they expect the highest standards from them.

A violet mother is the queen of the house and an excellent manager of a busy household. The violet father is a distinguished, cultured and generous man; a natural aristocrat.

A violet's home needs to provide a feeling of space and openness, with various *objet d'art*, old books and antique furniture creating a warm and distinguished atmosphere.

Violet children are gentle and sensitive, prone to being over-protected by their parents; they may have high energy levels and be fidgety at school. They want to enjoy life to the full. They need to be left alone to find their way through life and to be encouraged to be considerate and charitable – as it is very natural for a violet child to demand attention and material goods or to be lazy. Violet children should be encouraged to share their gifts and abilities with the rest of the world.

At work

Positive violets exude calm energy, and appear to be self-confident and in control. Their positive attitude and great respect for their colleagues bring the best out of others who wish to help and honour them.

Violets are gifted, dignified and usually very knowledgeable and cultured people open to all subjects, from the stock market to the metaphysical. They are excellent bosses who will bring their company to great heights, always keeping their employees' needs in their minds. It is not unusual to find violets chairing big charities or companies that make the world a better place.

Violets can be found in the artistic world, playing or conducting music, reading poetry, reciting Shakespeare or bringing their newly inspired productions to the stage or screen. Violets can also excel in many different fields; they are often multitalented. Many therapists, psychic readers and clairvoyants are violet personalities.

How best to handle violets

It is important to remember that violet personalities are pleasure oriented. They need to feel that things have been made pleasant for them, so that they will comply with the wishes of any individual.

Violets have bountiful energy that all other colour personalities can tap into, so violets can teach us how pleasurable life can be. Remind them how joyful life is and how much their generosity is appreciated.

Negative violets are totally out of control and dominated by their impulses. To support the violet personality, help them to find a commitment in their lives, to become experts in a particular field, and encourage commitment to one relationship; only then will they be able to reach their full and wonderful potential.

Helpful hints when things get tough

Violet personalities need to make life pleasurable, fun and adventurous. With a good set of rules around them, they will be happy to try hard to achieve their goals. They need to understand that for good things to come their way, a certain amount of effort is essential.

Violet affirmation

All life is sacred. The pleasure is in the journey itself

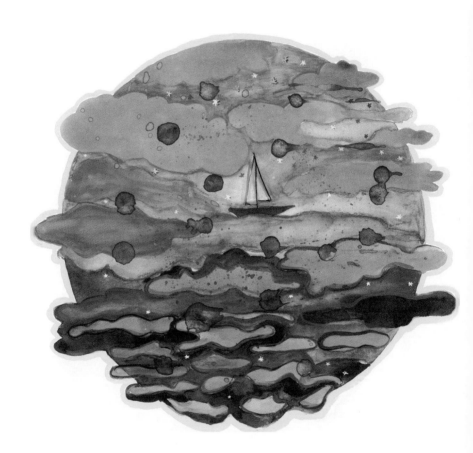

MAGENTA personality

Life goal: self-transformation / **Life gift**: fearlessness

General traits

Magentas can be dreamy and have fertile imaginations with many creative instincts – not just artistic but business-wise as well. Magentas make great entrepreneurs and business people, and can attract abundance with their bountiful luck. All this dreamy, heavenly energy means that sometimes magentas don't want to come back to earth and would prefer to stay in the clouds, getting lost in spiritual dreams.

The main ambition of a magenta is to serve and protect others, and they spend their life working at being the right leader. Magentas can feel at home anywhere in the world. Because of their expansive energy they tend to build relationships with overseas organisations and individuals immersing themselves in exotic cultures. If they choose not to travel physically, then it is travel of the mind – spiritual and emotional quests – that becomes very exciting.

Magentas pride themselves on their good taste, and surround themselves with beauty and attractive objects. Although they are not solely concerned with material wealth, they love what they can afford, and are pleased when they have items of beauty in their homes or offices.

Magenta personalities are fantastic at organising events, projects and parties for both business and pleasure. They have a high degree of maturity and understanding about the world, and are able to deal with life's challenges and obstacles with compassion and gentleness. Magentas are also cheerful and happy when in a social environment, and they have great energy that attracts even more company.

Magentas are kind. They are connected to the universal energy of divine love, and just being around them helps other individuals to release and let go of anything that is holding them back.

Sometimes, magentas can seem outrageous and shocking, but this is just the outcome of innovative new ideas arising from an extensive imagination. Magentas like to have many ideas and projects on the go: some they quickly drop, others they will continue to enjoy until they eventually complete them.

Magenta is the colour of negotiation, so magenta personalities are great to have around during a disagreement. They are capable of seeing both sides and negotiating a balance between common sense and practicality, creating win–win situations.

Magentas are spiritual but not religious – personal development is an important part of life for them. Religion holds too many boundaries for magentas, especially as unconditional love is one of the key values for this colour personality.

Pulling the 'rabbit out of the hat' as and when needed is a positive trait of magentas, and their resourcefulness is sought by many. Magentas are able to appreciate all that they have, and get great joy from the little things in life rather than the large and exotic.

Sometimes a magenta's sense of humour can seem a little weird and off beat, but they can laugh with others and enjoy the company of like-minded individuals.

Magentas dislike rules and regulations – although they are able to toe the line when required, they prefer to be free spirits. It is hard to tie them down, but they do like to have an organised life.

Magentas can also be over- or under-emotional, constantly striving for perfect balance.

Little issues consume magentas, which can make them needy and selfish, and may eventually create compulsive behaviours. They can also become rather arrogant and bossy, which can lead to a tendency to overwhelm and control.

Tricky traits

The constant drive of a magenta personality can lead to decisions being taken too impulsively, resulting in drama that could have been avoided if time and care had been taken in the first place.

This impulsive behaviour can lead to impatience and intolerance of many things. Sometimes, magentas will 'throw the baby out with the bath water', and have to start over (including, possibly, horrible behaviour towards loved ones).

This attitude can make magentas overbearing and dominant, creating a very intense personal style, with intolerance of others' taste and behaviour with no interest in their lives. They may enjoy humiliating, punishing and degrading others.

A bossy magenta is truly a nightmare for anyone around them: they can become so obsessed with the small things in life that they become needy, selfish and even compulsive.

Health and well-being

Stress can sometimes be the downfall of magentas, as they tend to juggle lots of balls in their lives, and when overwhelmed they can become overstressed, resulting in headaches, indigestion and ulcers.

Depression may sometimes affect magentas, because they try to balance physical, emotional, mental and spiritual needs all at once, and this can become too much.

As magentas are naturally compassionate, they are very susceptible to negative energies, and can be affected by them without even realising.

Adding sport to a magenta's agenda will help to balance the large amount of energy that they can expend. Dancing, aerobics and other body work-outs can help with relaxation and balance.

In the bedroom

Sex is all about harmony and love, and magentas are looking for a perfect balance in these attributes. The perfect partner for a magenta will love unconditionally and encourage gentle love-making so they feel fulfilled on four levels – physically, emotionally, mentally and spiritually. No pushy or coercing tactics should be used with magentas, but a good sense of humour and innovation will make love-making intense and exciting.

Sex for a magenta does not have to stay in the bedroom – a little spontaneous, outrageous sex, perhaps outdoors, in public, by the sea, in a car are all fun (not all at the same time!), fulfils a magenta's free spirit nature. Sex is a favourite activity that releases a magenta's vibrant energy.

Lingerie, silk sheets, crispy white cotton, luxurious throws of velvet, and smells to match, make the magenta bedroom very exciting. Surrounded by beautiful things that are visual allows magentas to enjoy sexual chemistry even more. Book a boutique hotel in a romantic setting, with champagne in the room, and magentas, both male and female, will feel at home.

When magentas are not feeling sexy or find their partner unattractive, then sex stops all together. Like most things in a magenta's life, it is about finding balance in everything that they experience.

In the family

Loving and affectionate, magenta parents bring cheerfulness and happiness into any family. They will do anything to protect their family and home. They are great at negotiating with other members of the family, and love organising events for family and friends, where they will add their own *soupçon* of unusual entertainment.

Bringing balance into the family with unconditional love and non-judgement is an area that magentas are renowned for. They see all points of view when there is an argument, and will make a fair and decisive decision about any misunderstandings, using their compassion and gentle energy.

If they become domineering and arrogant, then a magenta parent can be very hard work for their child. Living up to this parent's high expectations and their obsessive and often violent tendencies may be extremely difficult.

A magenta child will be loving and very expressive with his or her free spirit. If it is a girl, then the 'princess' of the house will make herself known very early on, and may also have a gang of imaginary friends whom she feeds, teaches and tells exactly what to do.

Magenta kids will be bright with distinct personalities, and will dislike rules. They will have to learn, though, that without rules they are unable to get what they require from life.

At work

When balanced, magentas make good managers – they can be happy, content and show appreciation for what has been achieved. They are able to adapt and change quickly, and as their energy is transformational they can release old patterns of working and create new and innovative ideas and procedures.

Magentas work best when they are inspiring others, so an artistic or creative pursuit is closely linked with this personality colour. Film, art, television – anything that is not contained or confined – will catch a magenta's eye.

Magentas have a great deal of common sense and can also be very practical, so you may also find them working in, for example, the computer industry, creating new and innovative games and applications. Magentas can sell anything that they love, as they want everyone to own what they have as well. Great sales people, they can make organisations plenty of money.

However, if a magenta becomes unbalanced, then they can turn into a domineering, pushy and difficult boss for a team.

You will often find items of beauty and art – which this colour personality find pleasing – in a magenta's office, and although they are not concerned with material wealth, they like what it can bring them, so magentas will always look for well-paid jobs.

How best to handle magentas

Ask a magenta about their opinion on something going on in the world and they will be happy to give you their thoughts with compassion and maturity. Ask them about art, sculpture, religion or any other subject that especially interests them, and you will instantly get them talking with you.

Humour and fun will help lift any heaviness from a magenta and make them smile with you. With magentas, patience is a virtue, and sometimes it is better to back off than to try to sort out any of their problems on their behalf.

Personal growth is important to magentas, so ask them about personal matters, where there will be positive answers allowing them to let go of old belief patterns.

Helpful hints when things get tough

When anxiety and the pressures of life are too strong for a magenta, then allow space for relaxation and just being. A walk by the sea or in the country can bring magentas back into focus.

Meditation and spiritual healing are great for magentas, allowing them to take themselves off on a journey of discovery before returning earth!

Magenta affirmation

Everything is exactly what it is. I am relaxed, I am open, I am present

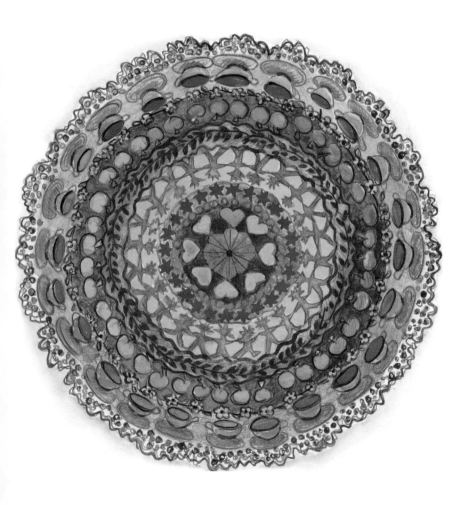

GOLD personality

Life goal: self-realisation / **Life gift**: equanimity

General traits

Gold personalities are humanitarians who wish to save the world; their ambition is to serve others. They are here to see godliness beneath reality; to see good in every event and in every person.

Golds are very old souls and therefore gifted with psychic abilities, guided by their higher selves. They are intrigued by the paranormal because they have great insight and innate psychic power. Their luminous personality lifts spirits up, as they exude an aura of optimism around them.

Teaching is natural for golds, and whether they do this professionally or not, they will find themselves imparting relevant information to others. They feel they have a mission to let people know that they are highly spiritual beings, full of power and unconditional love. They want to save the planet and its occupants from self-destruction, sometimes becoming martyrs to the world. In their purest form they are like beacons of clear light.

Golds may be missionaries and visionaries, perhaps fighting for the spiritual growth of underdeveloped countries. They like to share their knowledge and experience to help mankind grow and at the same time understand the meaning of life. They do not feel the need to be acknowledged, and often work behind the scenes, but accomplish a lot – they are benevolent, kind, giving and sharing.

Golds appear to have no aggressive drives, but in truth they repress these drives in order to create pleasant inner feelings and harmonious relationships. Peace, sometimes at any price, is what they thrive on.

Gold personalities like big spaces and luxurious things around them; with exquisite taste and talent, they create beautiful environments, open for everybody to admire and enjoy. When golds are truly switched on to their higher self, they take loving action to create a healing and harmonious environment for themselves and others.

Golds are here to serve and make the world a better place. They are good natured, easy-going, optimistic, unpretentious, reassuring and supportive; really nice people.

However, gold personalities can be too trustful, and by giving unconditionally they can easily become victims of unwanted situations. Their extra-sensitive nature means that they are easily offended, and they do not forgive easily. Although golds seem to exist for the good of the world, sometimes they lack energy and suffer from bouts of laziness, preventing them from working to achieve their ambitions.

A gold's wish is to be at a high spiritual level, and they will go to self-development classes, perhaps to learn meditation or yoga, but they can neglect to undertake the hard work of confronting and facing their ego and its deficiencies. Sometimes, it all seems to be too much trouble, and golds often wish that everything would continue on its own and let them be. In this case, golds will procrastinate or ignore a problem as long as possible, and hope others will take over their chores and tasks; they may even daydream of someone else doing their job!

Gold contains all the colours of the spectrum; in a similar way, gold personalities have characteristics of all the other colours. This makes them resonate at ease with all the other colour personalities, to merge with them and internalise their perspectives. They give others a sense of being understood and validated.

Tricky traits

On the surface, gold personalities seem quite easy-going, agreeable and adaptable. They are friendly and do not seem to mind going along with the wishes of others, but at a deeper level, golds do not want to be made to change, or to be other than who and what they are already comfortable with.

Golds can seek to keep themselves oblivious in order to avoid facing reality; they procrastinate, certain that the problem will disappear if ignored.

Negative gold personalities may have a tendency towards possessiveness, neurosis, conceit and volatility. They may be impulse buyers. Promiscuity can be a problem for them because they are constantly pursued because of their magnetism, and they do enjoy flattery. They may have false expectations and a fear of being alive.

Health and well-being

Gold personalities need to be well connected with their mission in life in order to be balanced and healthy; they need to be in touch with their higher self, and in order to achieve this state it is highly recommended for them to spend time around their home and in their garden, where there is beauty, peace and serenity.

Golds need to be surrounded by their favourite, often luxurious, objects. They also need to look after their body and to keep it clear of toxins; the clearer the body, the purer the light that shines through it. Harmony, peace and safety are all important to the well-being of the gold personality.

The life goal of a gold personality is to bring light, love, compassion, service and connection with higher values into the world. It is very important for golds to keep their energy open and clear, and if they spend too long in crowded places or dealing with challenging people, they need to regain their balance and purity – through yoga, meditation and other holistic exercises.

The colour gold corresponds to the kidneys and generative organs, and also to diseases that are hard to diagnose and brought about by self-indulgence and unhealthy habits. Alcohol and drugs are taboo for gold personalities. Good health depends upon having their feet on the ground and adopting good living habits. Not facing reality can be their undoing.

In the bedroom

Golds tend to attract problematic people in their intimate relationships, in the hope that by loving and caring for them they can heal hurts.

The natural generosity of golds follows them in the bedroom, where they will do anything to please their lover. Because they are so trustful, they will abandon their hearts and their bodies to grant all their partner's wishes.

Gold personalities have a kind of innocence that makes them sexually irresistible; nudity is one way to become closer to our inner selves, and golds feel totally at home in their birthday suit!

Love-making can be the highest form of union for golds, which is something they wish for earnestly, and go after again and again. Sex is important for a balanced gold.

A beautifully decorated, spacious bedroom full of sunshine is a gold's ideal love sanctuary. With candles, scents and lush, soft, textured linen, they can reach ecstasies of feeling. Tantric sex is recommended for the more spiritually developed golds.

In the family

Gold personalities will create a beautiful home for themselves and their families. They are usually content with life as it is; they are emotional anchors providing a stable, loving presence. Wonderful in their parenting, they have no limits to their generosity in time, love and money for their children. They believe that everything is possible, and will never criticise negatively in problematic situations. They are the most trustful personalities of all: they trust themselves, they trust others and they trust life.

A gold's great optimism will allow them to pardon everyone and everything, but they need to learn to double-check things and not to always trust unconditionally.

The capacity of golds to mix well with other people makes them excellent mediators and parents. They can see all sides, and they have all the patience in the world to solve problems, always finding something good in everyone. They do not have anxieties because they have faith that they will be looked after and provided for from above. They really do bless the bad with the good. Their ability to see this truth makes then genuinely inspired and inspiring parents.

When gold personalities are not at full strength, in order to preserve the peace they will agree with everyone's point of view, trying to please everybody but pleasing no-one in the end. At low ebb, golds want peace at any cost.

Gold children need good guidelines to protect them against bullying, or being taken advantage of. Pay attention to them, ask their opinion, inquire after their needs; this will make gold children feel loved and willing to confront conflicts they would otherwise flee from.

At work

Gold personalities are quiet but not passive; many are ambitious. When they are in a leadership position, they rule in a strong but gentle manner that wins everyone's confidence. They have a special warmth that makes everybody feel that they are cared for as individuals. Their great faith that all is predesigned from above makes them trusting, gives them strength and inspires them to provide guidance.

However, golds can lose control by refusing to face reality and by allowing things to happen simply to keep the peace. Their partner or a friend should help them see what's right and wrong. A partner can also help to stimulate a gold's enthusiasm: some golds tend, at times, to wait for things to happen 'magically' without their making any effort whatsoever!

Golds are pleasant to have around at a work because of their optimistic and cheerful presence. They exude a wonderful light that uplifts people's spirits.

How best to handle golds

Ask a gold their opinion, and help them by paying attention to them and expressing appreciation. Enquire after their needs. This will make them feel loved, which in turn makes them more attentive, confident and willing to face conflicts that they would otherwise flee from.

Help golds by giving them a chance to serve and to be of service to themselves.

Helpful hints when things get tough

Golds need love and affection. When love is the higher state of a gold personality, they become carriers of deep compassion, nobility and unshakable inner peace. Being dynamically awake to every moment, the ideal gold personality is moved to achieve peace and harmony and awareness of the dynamic unity of existence.

Golds can be too naive and trusting, and can end up in awkward situations. They need to be a bit more realistic about life, and not take everything at face value.

Gold affirmation

Not only am I loved, I am actually made of love

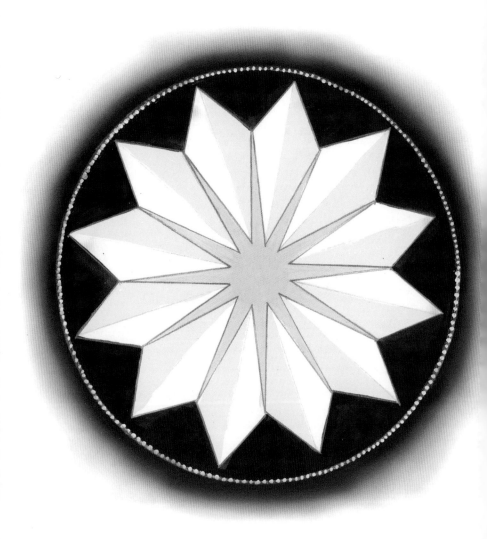

PART 2
Your journey colours

Welcome to the second part of the book, which adds further unique and in-depth information to the colour personality by looking at the individual colours of the day, month and year of birth. These three colours create the individual's signature or unique colour chart along with the nine colour personalities.

These are either known as 'supportive' colours or 'journey' colours, as they are relate to childhood behaviour, day-to-day skills and life aspirations. The ancient races believed in reincarnation, and colour is a tool that can change depending upon required experiences in each life journey.

Interpreting and consciously applying the qualities of our day's, month's and year's colours will give us tools that we can use to grow and develop into the best of ourselves through our life's journey.

Do endeavour to dig deeper into this section by getting to know the qualities of your unique colours and how they can support you on a day-to-day basis.

The colour of the day: our inner child

The numeric day of your birth corresponds to a colour. If this number is above 9, add the numerals together, to give a number from 1 to 9. For example, if you came into this world on the 23rd of the month, you add the 2 to the 3 to get 5, and 5 = blue:

23 = 2 + 3 = 5 = blue

1 = Red	4 = Green	7 = Violet
2 = Orange	5 = Blue	8 = Magenta
3 = Yellow	6 = Indigo	9 = Gold

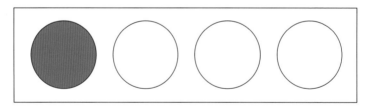

The first colour from the day of birth relates to the 'inner child'. The inner-child qualities tend to be strongly displayed from birth through to approximately 9 years of age.

A 'care free' childhood permitting freedom of expression and where 'just being yourself' was allowed and honoured shows the positive qualities of this colour. The day's colour may be as dominant as the colour personality, so it is important to fully understand its qualities.

If a child's upbringing was one of control and strictly enforced rules and regulations, the inner child's qualities may be suppressed. It is then more difficult to recognise and to acknowledge the qualities of the inner child's colour. It can also be depleted by different influences and conditioning during our life's journey. It is always worth revisiting our inner child.

Our connection with this first colour relates very much to our essence. If there are issues that need to be healed, they often stem from childhood. Revisiting this time of life and understanding the qualities of the colour may help to resolve early traumas.

The inner child is always within us – bright and as pure as the very early years of life. So many wonderful qualities that might have become forgotten due to life's conditioning or the fear of who we really are can be rediscovered by tapping into this colour, helping to enrich the colour personality.

Work on boosting the positive qualities and on managing the less beneficial ones. Slowly, these positive qualities will emerge naturally and be reactivated in daily behaviour. Listen to the inner child's way of viewing the world in its inborn wisdom.

The inner child comes to the forefront when life is joyful and not taken quite so seriously; freedom and happiness are very important parts of life.

It is also very valuable for parents to understand this colour in their children and to see how their personalities will develop as the years unfold. A strategy can be developed to support and guide their offspring along a constructive path using the power of the colour of the inner child and its language – which is both positive and forward thinking.

Combining the inner child's colours – whether warm (red, orange and yellow), balanced (green), cool (blue, indigo and violet) or 'bigger picture' (magenta and gold) – can either increase the strength of the personality or decrease its intensity.

The colour of the month: skills

From the numeric month of your birth, add the numerals together to give a number from 1 to 9 corresponding to a colour. For example, if your month of birth is November (the 11th month), this relates to the number

11 = 1 + 1 = 2 = orange

1 = Red	4 = Green	7 = Violet
2 = Orange	5 = Blue	8 = Magenta
3 = Yellow	6 = Indigo	9 = Gold

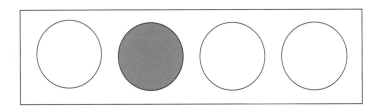

The qualities of the month's colour are used as a guide to day-to-day behaviour. The colour's qualities reflect the skills and abilities that are part of an individual's natural talents. Using these qualities in your life is a fabulous tool to turn challenges into success stories.

The month's colour represents innate natural talents. By connecting and identifying with them, a smoother journey is guaranteed.

Honouring personal skills and constantly improving them brings peace of mind.

The month's colour can give information on careers and job choices, supporting the colour personality. It also shows how creativity and communication are experienced. The warmer colours (red, orange and yellow) demand action and are more reactive. The cooler colours (blue, indigo and violet) are more observing and taking a step back prior to decision making. The balance colour (green) needs steadiness and the bigger-picture colours (magenta and gold) require the faith to go with the flow.

Skills and talents are also important in romance and love relationships. The biggest problem in relationships is that we all behave differently, which can cause confusion and misunderstandings. Knowing the month's colour leads to a better understanding of how behaviour may be expressed. So, this information alone can completely transform a relationship and create a happy outcome.

When dealing with children, the month's colour gives information about how to approach them, helping them with decision making, getting them to understand their behaviour in line with their colour personality. This will make their life journey easier and less stressful, bringing confidence, since we will have a fuller realisation of who they really are and how they should act.

The colour of the year: aspirations

Take your year of birth and add the four numerals together until you get a single number between 1 and 9 corresponding to a colour. For example:

1975 = 1 + 9 + 7 + 5 = 22 = 2 + 2 = 4 = green

1 = Red	4 = Green	7 = Violet
2 = Orange	5 = Blue	8 = Magenta
3 = Yellow	6 = Indigo	9 = Gold

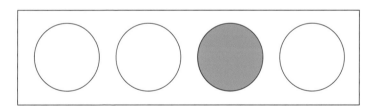

Understanding the qualities of this colour brings an awareness of your life's purpose. The year's colour provides an opportunity to understand and experience the lessons of this journey.

Career and job roles that are unfulfilling may not include these characteristics that are so important for self-realisation. Acting upon the qualities of this colour can give direction, confidence and knowledge throughout the journey, ensuring that the right path is being chosen.

The colour of aspiration is equally as crucial for relationships – whether with your partner, family, friends or colleagues. Once the goals of our aspiration colour are set, it has the potential to attract healthy interaction and behaviour in all relationships.

When we ask ourselves, 'What is my life's purpose? What am I here for?', the answers are waiting to be found in the many qualities of the year's colour. Study those qualities, eternalise them, express them not only in daily behaviour but through different creative ways such as writing, singing, dancing, doodling or storytelling. Meditate upon them: find their accurate meaning in a dictionary, check how they sound in different languages (Latin can have a revealing effect), explore their roots, and see how they appear in literature and other media. Resonating with the qualities of the year's colour is the path to self-realisation.

Have you calculated the colours your day, month and year of birth? Check your calculations – it's important to get the numbers correct.

People with warm colours (red, orange and yellow) need to learn and experience by 'doing' and creating. Those with the balance colour (green) require harmony and stability through a peaceful environment. Those with cool colours (blue, indigo and violet) need to express and develop intuition and communication. Individuals with bigger-picture colours (magenta and gold) need to experience universal flow in body, mind and spirit.

Now, turn the page to begin your fascinating and life-changing colour journey …

How your journey colours support your colour personality

Helpful colour theory: for a more profound understanding of the qualities of colours

Colour is energy, which can be measured in wavelengths and frequencies. The colours that the human eye can see cover only a tiny part of the electromagnetic spectrum. What you see in the diagram opposite are the visible colours: all the other energy is not visible to the human eye, but some can be felt, like heat (infrared).

The visible spectrum is between 4×10^{-7} and 7×10^{-7} metres in the diagram (or, more conveniently, 400 and 700 nanometres). Each colour is defined by its frequency and wavelength. As a rule of thumb, long wavelengths have low frequencies, while short wavelengths have high frequencies.

Low-frequency, long-wavelength colours (towards the red end of the spectrum) have less energy than high-frequency, short-wavelength colours (towards the blue end of the spectrum). However, red light is closer to the energy of the molecules in our bodies, so, from the viewpoint of colour therapy, it is perceived as more energetic than blue light.

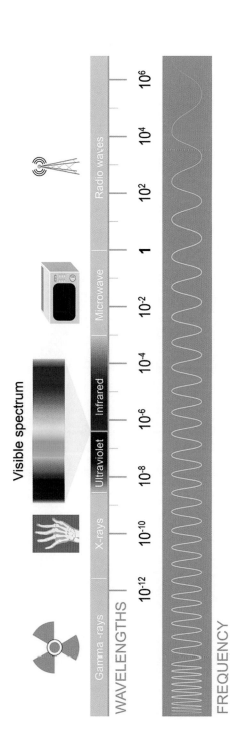

The electromagnetic spectrum

103

Applying this theory to colour personalities, people with warm colours tend to be more intense, busy and easy to read. People with cool colour personalities prefer to be less intense; they observe and tend to hold back. Green sits in the middle of the spectrum and has both warm and cool qualities, and therefore people with a green personality tend to have restoring and balancing properties.

According to one colour system (the subtractive set of colours, often used for paints and other pigments) there are three primary colours and three secondary colours. Red, yellow and blue are primary and pure. Orange, green and violet are secondary, and derive when two primary colours are mixed together in equal amounts. Primary colours are more intense than the secondary colours.

Each primary colour has a secondary colour as its complementary: red and green, yellow and violet, blue and orange.

Other colours are mixtures of unequal amounts of primary colours: for example, magenta is a mix of two parts red and one part blue, creating its negotiating qualities. Gold is made up many combinations of colours; it is used to describe light which contains all the spectral colours. This is also reflected in that colour personality.

These mixed colours also have complementary colours: for example, lime green (one part yellow, two parts green) and magenta. White and black (which stand for light and darkness) are complementary too.

When reading your colour combinations, consider this information: it will give an even deeper insight into your own personal colour chart and your relationships.

RED as your journey colour

The colour of the day: your inner child

This vibrant colour is hot and fiery, with a great deal of energy. Your red inner child is anxious to try new things, to act instantly and fearlessly. You are always a bit impatient to get things moving; and have a kick in your step.

Your red inner child gives you courage from a young age. Of the inner child's colours, red in particular is capable of overcoming early childhood disappointments, illnesses and emotional challenges because of its fiery nature to consume quickly.

This colour grounds your body to the earth, connecting you to traditional qualities and thus giving you a touch of conservatism.

Young red children tend to demonstrate great levels of security in themselves, and can be direct and say exactly how things are.

Reacting forcefully to any situation is a strong quality of red, so try to calm down for a second or two, to become fully aware that it is the red energy that is pushing you to do things too fast. Doing a sport or channelling a physical interest will help young reds to disperse energy.

With a red inner child you could easily 'crash and burn', but you are able to pick yourself up again and start something new.

If this fiery energy is suppressed, then there could be physical challenges later in life.

In a nutshell, when red is your day's colour, you tend to:

- be busy with extra surges of energy – possibly slightly ADHD
- be traditional, looking at family roots
- be courageous and rise to any challenge – personal survival
- be outspoken and tell it how it is
- get bored easily
- need to have your own space and material things
- be insular and self-oriented.

The colour of the month: your skills

There is no doubt that reds are busy and do not procrastinate too much. You may be drawn to careers and jobs that mean that involve physical activities, such as sport, driving and sales. If you are not active in your daily role, then do make sure you have an outlet for your excess energy.

You are always able to complete your tasks, as you like to be efficient and productive. You can take a leadership role if you choose to do so, but it may be that you prefer your home life to a dynamic career. You don't lack courage, so if an opportunity arises that you can increase your income and independence, then take it: you are capable, and it will increase your confidence.

You may be drawn to organisations that create new technology, and like to be in a creative environment otherwise boredom may set in. Choose projects and tasks that ignite your passion and drive: you will stay interested and complete projects if they connect with this energy.

You feel better if your family structure is kept traditional and conservative. Create a family environment that suits you, but don't try to influence others too directly.

You like to be independent and are not too keen on authority although you will always adapt. So, ensure you make a space for yourself, and don't always rely on someone else.

In relationships, express your passion for someone quickly and openly and show that you desire them, but don't be too pushy.

In a nutshell, your journey will be smoother if you:

- are a doer – you get on with things, are physically active and don't procrastinate: *just do it*
- find a way to balance your excess energy
- choose a job/career with a varied role
- take a leading role, because you have the courage to do so
- choose projects and tasks that ignite your passion
- make space for yourself and don't always rely on someone else
- don't allow impatience to take over – it destroys what you have already created
- express your passion for someone quickly and openly.

If all else fails: *make love not war!*

The colour of the year: your aspirations

Red is such a vibrant and warm colour that it can frighten some people because of its physical power – but when used positively it is exciting and unpredictable.

The main quality of red is courage, and if you are an aspiring red, then courage is what you are learning about. You might have had to overcome adversities, having to pick yourself up and start again; this is common when year's colour is red.

Red also is associated with independence and initiative: you may have found yourself having to sort things out on your own or spending time alone. Red helps you to do this by giving you the physical strength along with emotional security to support you through these changes.

Being an aspiring red means that you need to just 'get on and do it'. Don't be afraid: there is nothing that you cannot overcome and, yes, at times it may be tough, but you can succeed, as this colour of drive and passion allows you to be motivated by change.

In a nutshell, you will get closer to completing your aspirations by:

- learning to be independent
- overcoming physical challenges
- having the courage to face adversity
- learning to love new beginnings – become excited about change and learning how to change
- feeling secure in yourself – become self-aware of the person that you truly are

- developing drive and passion in your life – you may be here for many years
- honouring your roots and traditions.

ORANGE as your journey colour

The colour of the day: your inner child

Orange is warm and joyful, just like a happy child. When you have this colour, you tend to have creative qualities, enjoying painting, dance, craftwork or anything that stimulates your ability to create something out of nothing.

Freedom is associated with this colour, and you do not like to be told what to do – maybe having a cheeky quip in return! Orange children are funny – clowning around, with a great sense of humour. This can turn into emotional demonstrations just as quickly, though, whether for drama or a spontaneous reaction to getting hurt, both physically and emotionally.

Your unconventional nature does not fit particularly well with structured environments – you prefer play and love interaction with friends. You can also become a little lazy when required to do something you don't enjoy.

Orange children are adventurous and love to take risks and will try anything, but sometimes do so without thinking of the consequences. Watch your food intake, even at a young age, as you may eat to suppress negative emotions.

In later life, your inner orange child adds a wild side to your personality: dig it out and indulge in its sense of humour. Life will be more fun when you allow the zany orange to manifest within you.

In a nutshell, when orange is the colour of your day you tend to:

- be spontaneously emotional – one minute crying, another laughing
- be creative – e.g. painting or dancing.
- have a great sense of humour, and be eccentric and wild.
- be caring (feminine element), and valuing relationships
- become lazy, or not bothered by norms (unconventional)
- not deal well with authority – you don't like to be told what to do
- be adventurous and a risk taker
- play the joker – clowning around and making fun of everything.

The colour of the month: your skills

People with orange skills are sociable and warm individuals who are adaptable and work exceptionally well as team players in a working environment. A creator of ideas and a great starter of projects, this orange energy brings to life new and stimulating opportunities.

You may even be a little eccentric, perhaps wearing unusual clothes, and are full of exuberance when you are excited about a project or person. You tend to choose non-conventional careers and '9 to 5' does not suit your personality, and may feel trapped by its limitations – freedom is of prime importance to you.

You may be a great cook, but do make sure that you share the food with those you love, as you may be someone who can over indulge.

As you are warm and sociable, you enjoy being around the family and hosting events at your home.

In one-to-one relationships you function better when both of you have the space and freedom to express your individualities. You don't want to be tied down to anyone or anything, but you tend to have emotional outbursts when your needs are not met.

To support your orange traits, make sure that you enhance your life by giving yourself the freedom to make decisions and use your creativity in fulfilling roles throughout your journey.

In a nutshell, your journey will be smoother if you:

- join in as a team player – stay sociable and warm
- go beyond the norm – use your eccentricity and exuberance for life
- expand your own horizons – don't choose '9 to 5'
- eat good food and make healthy choices
- create a fun and family-orientated environment and share your warmth
- create space at times just for you
- keep in check your emotions – don't overindulge your outbursts.

If all else fails: *take yourself to the dance floor!*

The colour of the year: your aspirations

If your year is orange then your aspiration is about allowing freedom to create the life you want. Letting go is also synonymous with this colour, and it may be that your challenge is to 'let go' of everything you know in your journey through life.

The creative element of life does not necessarily mean artistic – it could also refer to bringing to life new projects and designs that have not even been thought of yet. You may be able to start your own business, as this fits in with the non-conventional traits of this colour and is not '9 to 5'. You also have the talent to bring the best out of your team.

Freedom may also refer to relationships where you need to learn to 'let go' of the past – whether someone behaved well or badly. Learning that these emotions are deep and need clearing could be part of your journey.

In a nutshell, you will get closer to completing your aspirations by:

- being social, warm and adaptable – be part of a team even if you feel that you do not 'fit'.
- being creative and a 'birther' of exciting projects
- going beyond the norm with creative decision-making
- choosing a hobby that you love and making it a career – take the risk
- eating good food but watching your diet
- creating a family feeling in any situation and sharing your warmth
- keeping space for yourself and another in one-to-one relationships
- keep a check on your emotions and don't overindulge in outbursts.

YELLOW as your journey colour

The colour of the day: your inner child

Yellow is the colour of sunshine and brightness. When this colour appears as your inner child colour, then there is great clarity of mind. You may be very capable of learning new technologies quickly, and you have an aptitude towards study. You may have found that as a child you were attracted to Lego and Meccano and anything that stimulated your thinking processes.

Your yellow inner child tends to be good at decision-making even at an early age. When the young brain is not fed with negativity, a yellow child is able to adapt quickly to new processes and places. Smiling and a sunny disposition is so yellow inner child, but this can be extinguished easily if their upbringing is dull and controlled. Confidence tends to get knocked quite easily.

This colour also predisposes to acting or putting on a front, so yellow children tend to be able to turn their hand to various roles and play various roles. Enjoy playtime with a yellow child, and then remember this about yourself if your inner child is yellow: play makes the sunshine. To support this colour, add yellow to areas where children may study, to help develop their mental energy.

Take on small projects that interest you so that you can reconnect with your inner yellow. Make sure that you deal with your confidence issues by bringing positive values and people into your life.

In a nutshell, when yellow is your day's colour, you tend to be:

- sunny and not taking life too seriously – predominantly happy, uplifted and fidgety
- pretending to be different personalities – taking on different roles
- bright and mentally alert
- capable of thinking outside of the box
- in danger of overanalysing
- in need of a purpose.

The colour of the month: your skills

With yellow as your month's colour, you have a great need to be organised. You may keep 'to-do' or shopping lists. Ticking off the tasks is fulfilling and is a positive way for you to feel that you are achieving things.

You have a great ability to think outside of the box and come up with fantastic solutions to everyday problems. Do make sure that you keep focused on one thing at a time, though – too many 'lightbulb' moments can be very distracting!

You are gifted with being a connector of people as your networking skills are excellent. You have the capability of talking to anyone anywhere and introducing the right people to the most beneficial connections.

In a relationship, you are at your happiest when your intellect is stimulated, so you need a partner who connects with you at this level as well as other qualities. Sometimes though you can be too serious too quickly, and will overanalyse everything – just let go and have fun!

Connect with your spirituality: this will relax your crowded mind and help you to think outside of the box so that you can light a new way up for others.

In a nutshell, your journey will be smoother if you:

- use your impressive decision-making skills
- create a life plan with general outlines
- focus your energy on one thing at a time without too many novel ideas
- use your networking skills to manage groups and workshops
- don't allow negative self-confidence to affect you
- take life with a pinch of salt – don't overanalyse.

If all else fails: *go for a massage!*

The colour of the year: your aspirations

The connection between the mind and the body is an amazing tool, and aspiring yellows work hard to understand this connection during their life's journey.

Yellow people tend to overanalyse, so take care not to allow the mind to totally overrule the emotions and more spiritual aspects of your life.

An ongoing need to know how things work and a yearning for knowledge is also very much part of what you are here to learn. Yellow is fantastic for feeling and behaving younger, and your looks may also reflect the 'light' that this colour brings the older you become.

You must have your intellect stimulated otherwise you will find life moves by very slowly and tend to have 'sour' feelings for those that cannot keep up with you.

In a nutshell, you will get closer to completing your aspirations by:

- using your intellect when making decisions
- becoming organised – having lists and targets to achieve
- focusing your energy on one thing at a time – but not too many 'lightbulb' moments
- using your analytical mind to bring balance in all areas of your life
- using your communication and networking skills to bring people together
- making sure you share your world with intellectually stimulating people
- avoiding unnecessary anxiety by boosting your confidence and self-esteem
- not becoming over critical, as you can make your life 'sour'.

GREEN as your journey colour

The colour of the day: your inner child

Because green is found in the middle of the rainbow, making the transition from the warm colours to the cold ones smooth, it is a strong balancing colour.

Green is what enables us to breathe and to expand our lungs and our personality. If your inner child is born under rays of green, try to remember that you view the world straight from the heart without any filters of logic or wisdom.

Your inner child is gifted with a great sensitivity and able to feel things at a very deep level. Inner green children can be traumatised for life if they spend their early years in disharmony and hatred; they will need a lot of compassion, harmony and acceptance to allow their heart to trust that beauty and love can exist.

Don't be fooled by appearances of a strong personality if the colour of someone's day is green. Always approach this person with a warm, pure and compassionate smile.

To help a green inner child to blossom, create a beautiful and harmonious environment where they have an opportunity to care for something, like a pet or a special plant, or a family of dolls. Be tactful in the way you address the green inner child, as they are very easily insulted, and this eventually destroys their self-confidence.

In a nutshell, when green is your day's colour, you tend to be:

- loving, caring and compassionate
- extremely sensitive and therefore easily offended
- needing to belong to and be part of a community or family
- dexterous with your hands
- desirous to be outdoors
- mean and can be a little cruel
- prone to jealously – constantly comparing yourself with others (in search of balance)
- a procrastinator and stubborn – born out of the need to keep the balance.

The colour of the month: your skills

When your skills are green, many of your decisions come from your heart, meaning that you feel deeply about what is right and wrong.

Spending time in nature and being outside are extremely important to you. Breathing deeply and expanding your lungs allow you to relax. You have a great capacity to attract abundance, so do share this with those you love – you will receive love tenfold in return.

You have the capacity to stand back from other people's feelings, making you great in a crisis and in any career that deals with care of others.

When you are unhappy in your significant relationships you find it challenging to make the changes that are needed, as balance is of paramount importance.

In a nutshell, life will be smoother if you:

- follow your heart – your best decisions come from the heart
- take time to consciously breath and expand your lungs
- surround yourself with plants and pets, and spend time in nature
- nurture yourself – this is important for a harmonious balance
- share the abundance that you naturally create
- remember that your need to belong is important to your well-being
- are aware that your need to be always balanced can be overwhelming and could lead to stubbornness and procrastination
- know that you can step back when you are unhappy.

If all else fails: *wait for a lightning bolt!*

The colour of the year: your aspirations

Green rules the heart and is associated with self-love. When green is your aspiration colour, then you are working on getting to know and love yourself – faults and all.

When you are too overwhelmed by this colour, you step back from life. You need to build your own community network of friends and acquaintances that you support and nurture. This then reflects your own qualities, and you can see that you deserve to be loved.

The need for balance and harmony is also part of your learning the qualities of green. You may struggle with change, but expansion is what you are here to manifest. Healing is also a very strong drive for an aspiring green, and there are many individuals in the healing and medical world who were born in a green year. The heart energy from green is a powerful driver when considering a career in a healing profession, whether involving people, plants, animals or even the planet.

As an aspiring green, you may well be learning about how to make and handle money more effectively. Money is an exchange of services, so you may need to try your hand at selection of different careers before sticking to one chosen area.

In a nutshell, you will get closer to completing your aspirations by:

- learning to love yourself
- bringing beauty, peace and harmony around you
- becoming involved in some area of healing
- creating abundance in your life
- being compassionate – become part of a community
- learning to use your hands to create beautiful things or beautiful energies
- having an interest in environmental issues.

BLUE as your journey colour

The colour of the day: your inner child

Blue is a soothing receding colour that inspires trust and kindness. When your inner child is born under rays of blue, you will have the need to establish a private sanctuary all to yourself, where you can hide away from noisy crowds and indulge in your favourite occupation: broadening your knowledge.

Your inner child's blue will balance any exuberant fiery colours of your personality, but if the rest of your colours are in the blue end of the spectrum, you will tend to feel melancholic or slightly depressed. In this case, try consciously to divert your blue inner child's solitude or withdrawal by suggesting small charitable projects, especially when it includes others to help you feel good.

Listen to your inner blue child's needs with a very open mind and full acceptance, so that you gain trust. It is of the highest importance to know your inner child's truth, because this truth guides you throughout your life.

Gentle and kind, your inner child is easily hurt and can withdraw. The ability to communicate may be compromised if you are in negative situations during this early part of your life. When there is confidence, then your inner child can turn to 'nattering' and plenty of communication, preferably with adults – as this colour loves to learn from the grown-ups. Create a little haven for your inner child, either a private space or even a drawer that contains private things accessible only to the inner child.

Even as a young child the ability to be able to soothe and heal is present. Observation and listening are natural proficiencies, with the blue inner child standing you in good stead as you continue your life's journey.

In a nutshell, when blue is your day's colour, you tend to be:

- gentle, reserved and kind
- an observer and a little insular
- a natural healer (you can heal yourself)
- honest and direct, and thirsty for knowledge
- a little too concerned with your own health (learning difficulties)
- challenged in telling the truth
- in fear of rejection – leading to becoming a little manipulative.

The colour of the month: your skills

This gentle and kind colour can be very cool, and blues are known to be a great observers. The truth is sometimes hard to handle for people born in a blue month, so keeping feelings locked in is quite common for them.

Many types of work that require words suit you: marketing, writing, training and one-to-one communication. Healing is associated with this colour, and along with the gentleness and caring side that you possess, you might well find yourself in a carer's role.

You may sometimes be a little too direct for people, stating the truth exactly as it is. You find it difficult to 'smooze' individuals who you feel are untrustworthy. Your observation skills are excellent, though, and you will be able to feedback relevant information to all who need it.

In a personal relationship, you may struggle to ask for what you want, simply cutting off your connection from your partner if you are not happy. Your partner has feelings too, so make sure that you are using open-ended questions to allow the conversation to flow.

In a nutshell, life will be smoother if you:

- are in touch with your innermost truths
- communicate and express your feelings
- are kind – blue healing energy is always present, so try to incorporate it in your work
- are aware that you are efficient in crisis situations
- share your outstanding observation skills with other people – they can only benefit from them
- communicate your all-important truth with care and finesse, aware of other people's feelings
- prepare for two-way conversations in a relationship – use open-ended questions.

If all else fails: *don't sweat!*

The colour of the year: your aspirations

When you are an aspiring blue, the crux of your journey is to communicate your truths. Learn how to tell people around you what you want and why you want it. Your growth comes from your observation of others, but it is how you react to others that gives you the greatest understanding of life.

Trusting in your instincts and not shunning the opportunities to express yourself are clear qualities of this colour. The cool energy creates a feeling of detachment, but hiding away will not resolve anything. Your observations of the world around you are interesting and of value – make sure that you share the information with others.

If you harness the gentle and natural qualities of this colour, your ability to heal people with energy, observation and talking therapy will naturally increase. Be prepared to change your career direction if these qualities expand for you. Don't hide these skills away: the world is looking to be healed, and you can make a very valuable contribution.

In a nutshell, you will get closer to completing your aspirations by:

- finding and expressing your inner truths
- consciously expressing your inner world to those you trust
- supporting charities, helping the less fortunate
- creating a good health routine, and becoming involved in health projects
- creating a relatively structured career path – healing and supporting others

- surrendering any fears that no one can be relied on, and excepting that there is enough for everyone
- creating a life of variety around you to keep your heightened intellect challenged.

INDIGO as your journey colour

The colour of the day: your inner child

Indigo is the midnight sky's colour: deep, mysterious and absorbing. Being strong, disciplined and extremely intuitive, your antennae pick up things long before anybody else is aware. You will either be open to this energy and feel comfortable with it or lock it away forever if it scares you.

A natural ability of the indigo inner child is self-discipline, efficiency and devotion. There is, though, also a dose of fear around new challenges and situations. The ancient intuitive knowledge and wisdom that comes with this colour creates a slightly more reserved 'oomph' for life. The good thing is that your indigo inner child will always faithfully do its best to help you fulfil your plans and keep life in some sort of structure.

The intuitive side of this colour is extremely strong, and the need for justice means humanitarian activities (big or small) are a priority. It is of great value to organise little acts of kindness (towards animals or humans) for the indigo inner child: doing things for others will strengthen trust and alleviate any fear of the unknown   replacing them with love.

Your indigo inner child needs to hold your hand for comfort throughout your life: do provide it with unconditional love, patience and sincerity.

In a nutshell, when indigo is your day's colour, you tend to:

- naturally bring ancient wisdom to everyday life.
- be born with a highly developed sixth sense
- be 100% focused on what you decide to do
- give all of yourself – which can lead to a kind of addiction
- be a humanitarian, love animals, and want to save the world
- be fearful, with a tendency to pick up energies form other people
- thrive on routine – structured days, self-discipline, and love of law and order.

The colour of the month: your skills

With indigo as your month's colour, the need for structure is deepened on a day-to-day level. Jobs and careers are important, as they give a basis to your core personality. You may be attracted to organisations that are corporations or in the public sector, as there is safety and stability in there.

You have great ability to become an expert in your chosen subject or career. You clearly dedicate yourself to causes, whatever they may be, and you want to be the best.

You are also very good at helping the underdog. In situations that involve justice and fairness, you excel at supporting the individuals involved, and have a distinct view of how each person can gain from the outcomes.

Don't allow fear to stop you from spreading your wings. You have fantastic intuition, and when you focus it on a chosen subject it will bring clarity and understanding. Dream big, and you will be surprised by what you can achieve.

In a nutshell, life will be smoother if you:

- always use your amazing intuition
- find a job with a structured routine – you will feel safe and balanced
- know that anything that involves justice and fairness will attract you – this also applies to your friendships and relationships.
- make sure you that are efficient but also know when to say 'no'
- make sure that you are aware that you are naturally attracted to esoteric knowledge – don't let this scare you.
- remember, when drawn towards the underdog and helping others through trauma and neglect, to protect yourself from their chaotic energy
- promote yourself as an expert in the field – you have knowledge, so share it
- don't allow fear to stop you from dreaming big – take chances, and you might be surprised what you achieve.

If all else fails: *pray!*

The colour of the year: your aspirations

When indigo is your aspiration colour, it helps to bring structure and security into your life. Your intuition will be speaking to you every day: it is good to listen, so do not ignore it. The ancient knowledge that this colour brings connects you to deep and meaningful truths.

You may find yourself being drawn more and more towards the esoteric. Don't be afraid as your physic abilities deepen and you start to sense how people think, feel and communicate without having to speak to them.

This colour relates to an 'old soul': you are not necessarily old in age, but your understanding of life goes beyond what you have learnt in the 'here and now'. By connecting to this truth, you will find that there is nothing to fear, allowing you to spread your wings and experience all that life has to offer. Hiding away and fearing what may be can create feelings of depression and even lead to addiction if not kept in check. You have the skills to be an excellent teacher.

The depth of this colour brings an alternative edge to your life. You may think more deeply, become interested in meditation and want to expand your knowledge of subjects such as religions, new age concepts, new technologies and ancient pastimes. Enjoy this experience, as it will heighten your awareness of all that is.

In a nutshell, you will get closer to completing your aspirations by:

- developing your intuition and defining your inner values
- sharing your deep esoteric knowledge with others
- trusting that you are safe – have faith in what you do, and open up.
- working in a role that does good for the world
- developing your teaching – you are the perfect person for it
- understanding your fears and taming them
- living always with dignity and self-respect.

VIOLET as your journey colour

The colour of the day: your inner child

Violet has a high frequency, which lifts consciousness to higher levels. The violet inner child is extra-sensitive and very open to all kind of energies, which can strongly impact your delicate nature. You are both wise and perceptive but fragile and vulnerable too.

Fascinated and uplifted by life, you find yourself sometimes up and sometimes down. When you are influenced positively by cultural events, then your imagination flies. As you have a very sensitive inner child, do not overstress your body, as it reacts badly to tiredness, lack of sleep and poor nutrition.

Even at a young age violet people are very empathetic, and can find themselves affected by negative or difficult energies. Make sure that you protect yourself or you protect your inner child by using techniques that shield from these negativities (e.g. see yourself in a white bubble, protected from the world).

Night work is not an ideal for you, as your sensitives may react negatively to the lack of sleep and change in the circadian rhythms of the body.

In a nutshell, when violet is your day's colour, you tend to:

- have angelic energy – you live in your imagination
- are empathetic – you deeply understand both negative and positive feelings
- are charismatic in a noble way by supporting souls that need help
- balance between masculine and feminine – sometimes strong, other times weak
- be a drama queen (or king), and also a bit arrogant and bossy
- use manipulation in a constructive way
- have skin complaints and easily pick up illnesses due to your sensitive nature
- be a little naïve due to your overactive imagination.

Colour of the month: your skills

You are empathetic, which leads to an understanding of life from a more 'grey' perspective. You do not see life as 'black and white', 'good and evil'; instead, you tend to see the thin line between the two. You make a great councillor, and you attract individuals who need an ear. You may have a slightly addictive nature, as you can be attracted by a hedonistic lifestyle. Make sure that you have fun but don't get too carried away.

This colour offers leadership skills where leading comes from inspiration and innovation. The violet skills give you a visionary's touch, with the ability to conceive uncommonly big projects.

If you have spiritual pursuits, then violet as your month's colour means that your connections to esoteric knowledge are strong. You tend to attract that wonderful angelic energy that is gentle on the outside but strong and charismatic within.

Your strong feminine side means that you can listen and support people in all walks of life. Men with this colour tend to have a more feminine approach to life.

In a nutshell, life will be smoother if you:

- acknowledge your spiritual abilities and honour your connections
- use your empathetic skills in counselling situations but make sure you protect yourself
- always act with dignity and self-respect in a pleasurable way
- surround yourself with space and beauty
- help to resolve conflicts by equally balancing both party's perspective on situations
- connect with your feminine side whatever your gender
- be inspired – you receive information from any channelled sources – use it wisely
- don't let your hedonistic tendencies lead you astray – take the positive road

If all else fails: *host a dinner party!*

The colour of the year: your aspirations

With violet as your year's colour, you are looking to bring inspiration into your everyday life. With this colour, you are working with feminine energy – which is all about feelings and instinct.

Your connection with the more spiritual aspects of life tends to deepen, and you learn to understand how energies and the unknown play a part in our day-to-day life. You become sensitive to changes in the weather, moon cycles and even the moods of individuals in your vicinity.

An aspect of violet is that it can create hedonistic tendencies: be vigilant, but enjoy the freedom this gives.

Political tendencies grow strong with this colour. Making a difference in the world can become a very strong focus, so if you feel inspired to follow a political party, use the charisma that you have within you to influence those around you.

In a nutshell, you will get closer to completing your aspirations by:

- connecting closely with the spiritual realms for faith and inspiration
- developing your counselling skills and helping to resolve conflict
- connecting with your feminine side so that you can work comfortably with your feelings
- protecting yourself from negative people and situations
- using your charisma to charm and influence to help you succeed in business
- making sure that you take breaks and sleep well to keep your psyche in balance
- keeping on the right side of the road – don't get carried away by any hedonistic tendencies.

MAGENTA as your journey colour

The colour of the day: your inner child

Magenta is composed of two-thirds red and one-third blue. The red creates the fiery part of your early nature, but the blue allows you to be detached. This makes you a great negotiator, even at a very early age, leaving parents and teachers surprised by how often they have said 'yes'. The magenta inner child loves the stage and drama, and likes to be 'seen'.

Magenta energy constantly hovers between heaven and earth, and so, as a magenta inner child, you have an especially mercurial nature, constantly changing from a slightly cynical and grounded human being to the most gracious, enlightened angel. This duality provides you with extra coping abilities, but makes it a bit challenging for those around you who remain stuck in their earthy reality.

The ability to escape to an angelic realm will help the magenta inner child to see the world and yourself from a bird's eye view and get a better perspective of what reality is without involving personal judgement.

It is surprising just how much information you have incorporated from your early years, and you may find that you prefer the company of adults to children, as you feel more at home in their presence.

You are also related to a colour that is outside the body and in the aura, so you tend to be very grown up at an early age. Respect the magenta inner child's detached nature and allow escapism into the realms of magic. Storytelling, art and music strengthen this incorporeal refuge.

In a nutshell, when magenta is the colour of your inner child you tend to:

- have a strong and natural spirituality
- be grown up – understanding situations and issues from an early age
- be entrepreneurial at a young age
- be fearless and aware that change is a constant
- be detached, stepping to and from different places without spending much time in them
- be dominant as a child, as you like to boss others around due to your extensive knowledge of life.

The colour of the month: your skills

With magenta skills, you can constantly negotiate yourself into positive positions of power on a day-to-day basis. You really can get what you want: you weigh up situations and look for 'win–win' solutions.

You are very capable of 'going with the flow' by stating an intention and then allowing things to manifest on their own. You are fearless in the face of adversity, and will take on any challenge that comes your way. Make sure, though, that you understand that not everyone has your power – as this can sometimes make you very bossy and demonstrative.

You are entrepreneurial, and love the idea of running your own business. It is better that you are your own boss, as sometimes you cannot keep your temper when dealing with staff.

You have a keen eye for unusual and beautiful objects. So, your daytime role may include design or antiques. You can make money easily, but you can spend it readily too on anything that is beautiful.

In relationships, you need your freedom, and you can be a bit of a drama king/queen, so make sure that you have plenty of space. Tension can be created quickly, but also dissipate as quickly. You also can be 'off', quite literally, so do try to stay present with those around you.

In a nutshell, life will be smoother if you:

- go with the flow – state an intention, and allow things to develop in their own way
- remember that you are a change manager – your energy helps to reinvent projects with renewed interest
- are fearless in the face of adversity
- use your ability to detach from the decision-making process by taking the emotion out
- apply productivity in a supportive role to help others change
- keep your eye open for unusual and beautiful objects
- watch your tendency to live in a different dimension – stay present
- remember to share your generosity and fairness – bring joy and happiness

If all else fails: *meditate.*

The colour of the year: your aspirations

An aspiring magenta is looking to create 'win–win' situations in their life. You are wise enough to know how people 'tick', and you can use it to your advantage when you require support.

You are also learning about 'the bigger picture', looking at situations from a more holistic viewpoint. You may also become very interested in esoteric fields, along with heritage sites and anything that piques your interest in what has been here before.

Your tastes may have changed, and with magenta aspirations you are able to choose wisely, either for profit or just to sit elegantly in your own home.

You become more dynamic, maybe even venturing towards owning your own business and displaying your unique entrepreneurial abilities. Fearless in face of adversity is your mantra, so onwards and upwards towards success!

In a nutshell, you will get closer to completing your aspirations by:

- setting your intentions and letting the universe create your dreams
- applying your change management abilities to situations that require renewal
- using the blue part of your colour to detach sometimes – taking the emotion out

- developing your eye for antiques and bargains
- being generous with your time and energy – you will be rewarded with joy and happiness
- staying present – you might miss the things that are going on around you.

GOLD as your journey colour

The colour of the day: your inner child

Gold and white are interchangeable terms to define pure light energy, so as a gold inner child you combine all the colours of the spectrum. You also have the added quality of completion.

You were born wise: you know that you are here to experience life as a human being, and that one day when you have completed your experiences you will be going home again. This eternal knowledge makes your inner child bright and optimistic. No matter what happens in your life, your gold inner child constantly whispers to others that everything will turn out OK.

Gold, the colour of your inner child, has, strictly, been 'bestowed'. It displays moments of unconditional love for mankind. There tend to be no dark scary places for you – light illuminates the way. This does not mean that your life is easy – it just shows how flexible and positive you can be. Please your gold inner child by being trustful and allowing yourself to be vulnerable, making you fully open to life.

Treat your inner child with special pampering events, lovely holidays and uplifting conversations. Your Gold inner child can be a perfectionist and people-pleaser even at a young age. You need to be taught how to be trustful – but that does not mean being naïve and self-sacrificing.

The stronger your inner child's light shines, the better this world will be for you.

In a nutshell, when gold is your day's colour, you tend to:

- be extremely optimistic and wise
- be generous and easy-going
- have a straight connection to universal energies
- be a perfectionist – all must be 'just so' and done the 'right way'
- be lazy, expecting others to make things happen for you
- have a lust for money and material objects
- sacrifice your needs for a peaceful and unchallenging environment
- stay flexible and be an all-rounder.

The colour of the month: your skills

With gold as your skills colour, you have a great ability to oversee issues and decipher how the cause and effect of all situations will play out. Helping people is very important – not just caring but making sure that changes are made to bring better conditions to their everyday lives.

Your skills of completion allow you to see tasks and projects through to the end. Once you have started, then the chances are that you will finish, even if the outcome is not as fruitful as you had hoped. Always the optimist, you will see the good in all things and people, not taking sides but pointing out how each part fits together in the jigsaw of life.

Your flexible nature will flow through the challenges, and, as gold suggests, you can solidify and be rigid but also flow into areas that many others cannot even perceive. This may also be to do with your high connection to source. Your interest in religions, ancient histories and cultural pathways is heightened when gold is your skills colour.

In one-to-one relationships, you need to meet with a common connection, preferably spiritual. Endless discussions and hours sourcing information make your companionable nature easy to live with.

In a nutshell, life will be smoother if you:

- give without expecting to receive
- live and work with unconditional love
- be of service to all those that require your natural healing
- be optimistic – you are loved, and everything is OK
- know your ability to transfer information in many ways
- understand that a spiritual connection is important for a loving and lasting relationship.
- avoid being subservient – this can become a trait if not kept in check
- are aware not to step on other people in the hunt for material success.

If all else fails: *follow the light!*

The colour of the year: your aspirations

When gold is your aspiration colour, then you are learning about all aspects of unconditional love. You are also taking a completion journey – maybe you won't be visiting earth in the future as you have learnt a great many of your lessons. Your main lesson to learn is that you are loved and supported in every step of the way, from the day you came to this world.

You may also be learning about how not to put everyone first and finding some space for yourself, as unconditional love works for you too. You are here for service, whether that is helping your family and friends or a career role that supports others.

You are also finding your own natural way to express your knowledge and understanding of life. Your bigger-picture attitude allows you to see things from a loftier standpoint, taking in everyone's considerations and requests. Learning how to be flexible without giving in to everything is one of life's hardest lessons. Your journey this time makes that learning possible – enjoy the experience.

In a nutshell, you will get closer to completing your aspirations by:

- being of service – giving without expecting to receive
- loving unconditionally – supporting others in their time of need without judgement
- looking at things from a bird's eye view
- sharing your knowledge – finding new and interesting ways to distribute information
- working on being non-judgemental – seeing things from every perspective
- not victimising yourself and 'falling on your sword' for everyone
- being the light we are all made of.

PART 3
How to read colours

Tips on how to read colours

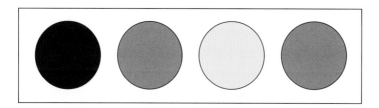

Look at your colours and decide how many are **warm** (red, orange, yellow), **cool** (blue, indigo, violet), **balance** (green) or **bigger issue** colours (magenta, gold).

This can indicate the following:

- How much of an extravert you are (**warm** and **bigger issue**).
- How much of an introvert you are (**cool** and **balance**).
- Your behaviour is predominantly busy and doing (**warm**).
- Your behaviour is predominantly observation (**cool**).
- You want to keep life on an even keel (**balance**).
- You seem to look at life from a bird's eye view (**bigger issue**).
- How balanced you are or could potentially be (**combination**).
- Where qualities of the colour are dominant (**inner child, skills, aspirations** or **colour personality**).
- How many double or triple colours you have.
- How many colours you and others have in common.
- How many colours you and your family have in common.

Double and triple colours

When colours appear twice or three times in a colour chart, then the colour is doubling or trebling its intensity. There is additional complexity where the colours reoccur, whether inner child and colour personality or aspirations and inner child.

The examples below give you an idea of how these combinations can work together to inform you further of your purpose and learning during your life's journey.

Double colours

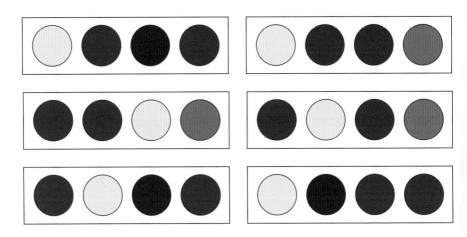

Inner child and skills: the qualities of the colour are required/ noticeable on a day-to-day basis.

Inner child and aspiration: the qualities of the colour may have not been accessed as a child and you are learning to reconnect with your inner child.

Inner child and personality: your experiences as a child are very connected to who you really are and how you express yourself.

Skills and aspirations: you are working hard to apply everything you know to fulfil your ambitions.

Skills and personality: your day-to-day behaviour is strongly connected to who you are and how you express yourself.

Aspirations and personality: your purpose in life is closely connected to how you express yourself.

Triple colours

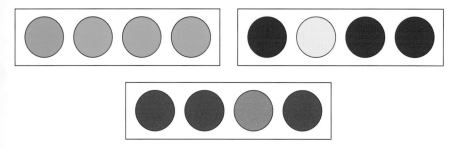

Inner child, skills and aspirations: high propensity to use the qualities of this colour throughout life's journey, e.g. learning to balance physical energy with the mental energy of yellow.

Skills, aspirations and colour personality: high propensity to use the qualities of this colour to overcome childhood issues.

Inner child, aspirations and colour personality: high propensity to ignore natural skills in favour of being seen to be someone different.

Quadruple colours

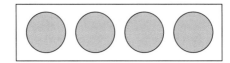

There is only one combination that has four colours, and this is gold.

When there are four golds, there is a strong desire to be of service to others and ignore your own needs. This combination has a strong sacrificial tendency, which could be expressed as chronic illnesses.

When this is out of balance, it can be displayed as an overinflated ego and a need for material success.

Example colour readings

How to use your colour knowledge

Queen Elizabeth and Prince Philip

Queen Elizabeth:
21/04/1926 = 3, 4, 9, 7 = yellow, green, gold, violet

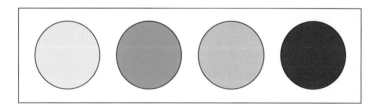

Inner child

Queen Elizabeth was born under yellow rays, which gifted her with clarity of mind, a certain amount of detachment, a need for freedom and originality. She has a natural understanding of how things work, and is attracted to science. She has an inborn light and a great love for people, whom she finds fascinating. With yellow's strength for networking, she can bring together the right people on the right occasions. Her inner child remains active – always busy and excited to be alive and discovering this wonderful world.

Skills

Her skills colour is green, which is the colour of balance, love and harmony. We can witness those qualities in the way she reigns: straight from the heart. Her mission is to preserve beauty, peace and harmony. She creates abundance in her world and shares its essence with the wider community (her kingdom).

Aspirations

Her aspiration is to learn gold's qualities: unconditional love, universal harmony, vital perfection, unconditional faith that we are all loved and that we all equally belong to a wider universe. Generosity, wisdom and abundance are also gold qualities. Gold is victorious and bountiful.

Colour personality

Her overall violet personality is that of a sovereign who reigns with dignity and self-respect, fully connected to her higher self for guidance and inspiration. With a violet personality, she is sensitive, with delicate health, gifted with the best social skills and the great ability to keep a conversation going about anything with anybody. Violet is a ruler through and through: caring for the community, leading with wisdom, thriving in art and culture, loving beautiful unique things and large, gorgeous places to live in!

Prince Philip:
01/06/1921 = 1, 6, 4, 2 = red, indigo, green, orange

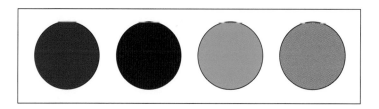

Inner child

Prince Philip was born under rays of red: he is gifted with courage, individualism, entrepreneurial skills and a solid connection to tradition and his roots. He acts spontaneously and quickly, always ready to confront any situation or challenge. His masculine side is strong and direct, loyal and always present.

Skills

His skills are indigo: they guide him to use his intuition for decision-making. Discipline, faith, loyalty, focus and efficiency are indigo's strongest qualities, which he needs to engage always, to protect and empower his queen. Indigo's qualities are also modesty, justice and a great sense of duty. By using his intuition, he can foresee challenging situations and people and act to prevent any possible troublesome behaviour.

Aspirations

His aspiration is to learn the green qualities, which are about self-love, harmony, beauty, peace, expansion, abundance and evolution. The green energy takes the hard edge of his red and indigo ones; it sculpts them into a work of beauty, love and comfort.

Colour personality

His overall colour is orange: that of a person who loves adventure, exploring and working with people to bring out their best qualities. He has orange's warmth, social skills and great sense of humour to brighten up any social gathering. With robust health and untiring energy, he can do anything and can be everywhere! He also has a creative and flamboyant side that inspires adaptability and playfulness

Their combined colours

Our Queen is a delicate and very bright violet personality ruled by the heart. She needs a strong hand to protect her from sacrificing everything for the common good. And this is where Philip comes in: his overall orange personality is fun, adaptable, warm and happy to be of service. He is a perfect match for his sensitive violet royal wife, who takes things deeply to heart and sometimes fusses unnecessarily. The jolly orange is there to lift her spirits up and to give her courage and faith to proceed with her work. Queen Elizabeth and Prince Philip share one colour (green) – the colour of the heart; together, they support each other to work untiringly, trying to establish love, peace, beauty, harmony and abundance in their kingdom.

David Beckham and Victoria Beckham

David Beckham:
02/05/1975 = 2, 5, 4, 2 = orange, blue, green, orange

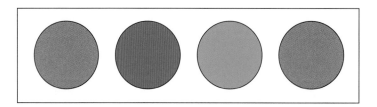

Inner child

David was born under orange rays: warm and funny, he is rather carefree and can sometimes be very much the practical joker. He filters this energy physically, which we can see in his career as a footballer. He was not just good at the sport, he excelled at it, creating opportunities for his team mates and setting up free kicks for others to convert. This reflects the creative ability of this colour. His occasional reported rows with his boss also reflect orange, as he does not like to be told what to do.

Skills

David's skills colour is blue, much cooler than the orange and giving him the ability to become a gentler individual and stand back and observe when the need arises. He was not particularly articulate at the start of his career but he has developed this skill to the point where people need to hear what he has to say.

Aspirations

His aspiration colour is green, so he is searching for balance and harmony in his life's journey. With this aspiration colour, he was also looking for love, and has found it within his family connections. Being the father of four children, he seems, from the press, to be deeply involved in their lives and contributes to their development. In recent pictures with his daughter Harper, you can clearly see his fatherly devotion.

Colour personality

His colour personality is orange, which gives additional energy to his inner child, which resonates in this colour. He is fun, has a great sense of humour and – I am sure – a practical joker. He is also very capable of showing his emotions, and makes an impact when working with young people needing support and help. As an orange, he fills his life with plenty of projects, allowing him to travel and enjoy an exceptionally fulfilled life.

Victoria Beckham:
17/04/1974 = 8, 4, 3, 6 = magenta, green, yellow, indigo

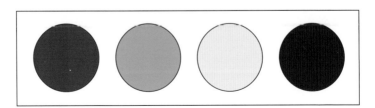

Inner child

Victoria was born under rays of magenta, so she was fearless and spontaneous from an early age. This is clear to see from her early life in the spotlight – a woman who enjoyed being seen. She clearly used her magenta energy to negotiate her place in the Spice Girls. Known as 'Posh', she portrayed herself as the most grown up of the group – a prominent quality of the colour magenta.

Skills

Her skills from green are displayed by having such a large family. Her kids mean everything to her, and although she has a career, the family comes first. Connecting with her sister and parents is as important to her as her children, and I expect her homes around the world are wonderfully decorated but with warm and comfortable surroundings.

Aspirations

She is an aspiring yellow, and so learning how to work with her mind and be original. Planning and organising fashion shows, she has been able to create a very successful unique business. The choice of fashion is yellow, as it is about how we look, what masks we wear and the enjoyment of dressing up. She is also learning about self-esteem, and although she appears confident, she may well be 'paddling hard' underneath the surface.

Colour personality

Her colour personality is indigo: deep and intuitive. This may be why we don't see her smile that often: indigo is cool. She loves structure and safety. She is the glue that holds together her family, keeping order and making sure all are safe and secure around her. She is very loyal, and would never think to have an affair, and she also works hard to earn her financial reward.

Their combined colours

Together, David and Victoria are opposites, as their colour personalities are orange and indigo: complementary colours. David's orange works well with Victoria's magenta, which at times can be strong. Both have green, so their actions come from the heart and they love each other and their family above anything else. They are also both connected with beauty and harmonious living.

All four colours

We are more unique than just our colour personality. In the language of colour and numerology we can offer a deeper insight into our life's journey by looking at our supporting colours from the day, month and year of our birth.

We will use the example from the beginning of the book to obtain this person's full colour chart, as follows:

Date of birth: 15/11/1965

15 = 1 + 5
  = 6
  = **indigo** – inner child colour

11 = 1 + 1
  = 2
  = **orange** – skills colour

1965 = 1 + 9 + 6 + 5
    = 21 = 2 + 1 = 3
    = **yellow** – aspirations colour

6 + 2 + 3 = 11
      = 1 + 1
      = 2
      = **orange** – colour personality

These colours are explained in detail in Part 2 of the book, with advice on how to create your amazing technicolour life.

Here is a blank chart for you to colour in, making it easier for you to visually see the colours of your life and those of your family, friends and colleagues.

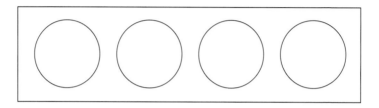

The Colour Ministry

Colour training

As natural healers, colour and light have many great qualities that can help your body heal naturally and give you a more positive psychological approach to life.

We offer workshops, including a one-day Colour Experience Workshop giving an overview of how colour and light can help benefit our world.

Our two-day Coaching Colours Workshop deals with the area of colour personalities and how to use colour to define who we are and how are relationships function from a colour perspective.

Our Diploma in Holistic Light and Colour Therapy is a nine-day certified course that is ideal for practitioners to complement their existing therapies or for those who are looking to delve into the fabulous world of colour healing.

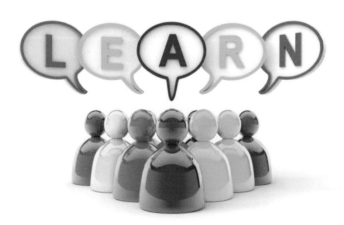

Visit our website at www.thecolourministry.co.uk, email Alison@thecolourministry.co.uk or phone +44 (0)1903 331234

Full personality readings

Having a Colour Personality Reading can give you inside information from a different perspective that can help enhance your relationships and make sense of some of those characteristics that you find challenging in relationships. Practical advice is also given on how you can positively enhance these relationships by adding colour into your environment.

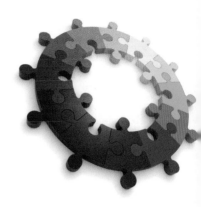

Colour Ministry membership programmes

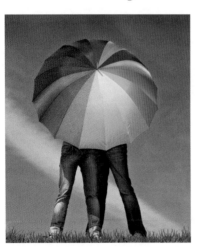

We offer a selection of membership programmes, which are a fabulous way to gain more insight into the amazing world of colour. These programmes run monthl with no contractual obligation. They are filled with invaluable information about your own colour personality and colour chart. They include written readings, birthday readings, colour products that support your colour personality, videos about the colour of the month, colour news and countless other benefits.

Visit our website at www.thecolourministry.co.uk, email Alison@thecolourministry.co.uk or phone +44 (0)1903 331234

Colour Discovery

Birthday colours picture

Finely woven threads create a unique composition with all four colours tailored to your personality, based on your date of birth. Below this charming composition, four cut-outs display the colours of the day, the month and the year of your birth and the core colour of your personality. A printed colour analysis of your personality accompanies each picture.

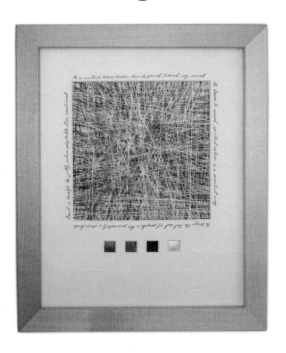

Define your life's purpose through colour

Our personality is affected by the qualities of the three colours we are born with. It is our third colour that defines our life's purpose: this class guides you in exploring the qualities of this colour in a creative, rewarding way through sketching, painting, writing and colouring. No experience necessary – all materials provided. See our website for next class date and location.

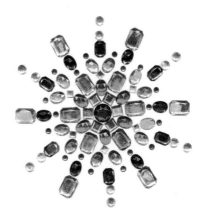

Visit our website at www.color-discovery.com, email theresa@color-discovery.com phone +44 (0)1273 303571

Colour therapy torch and treatment book

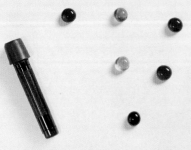

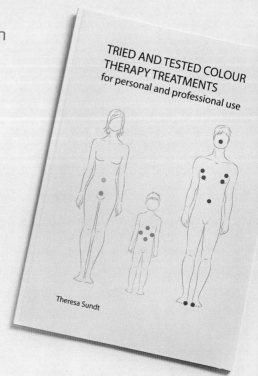

TRIED AND TESTED COLOUR THERAPY TREATMENTS
for personal and professional use

Theresa Sundt

Mainstream colour therapy for everybody, anytime and anywhere – easy to use and super-beneficial for our wellbeing. For personal and for professional use.

The Art of Colour Therapy

This book is an all-inclusive guide on how to use colour for healing and well-being. Through bright illustrations, visualisations and art projects, colour is experienced and enjoyed page after page. Read descriptions of each colour and learn about your unique colour personality.

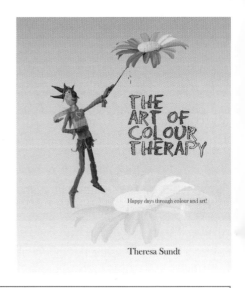

THE ART OF COLOUR THERAPY

Happy days through colour and art!

Theresa Sundt

Visit our website at www.color-discovery.com, email theresa@color-discovery.com phone +44 (0)1273 303571